Delusions of Grandeur

By Talmadge Rogalla

"One million people commit suicide every year"
World Health Organisation

Published by:
Chipmunka publishing
PO Box 6872
Brentwood
Essex
CM13 1ZT
United Kingdom

www.chipmunkapublishing.com

Introduction

This is a book of the thoughts going through a patient who is suffering from a psychosis. To my mind there is absolutely no other book that demonstrates this in view of 25 years of research. It is a gripping novel of the fantasies of a mind that has lost control of reality.

Frederick walks into a psychiatrist office and begins to tell his ordeal of what has happened to him at the hands of the Ministry of Defence when they extract information from him in order to save the world from nuclear devastation. Apollyon, an archangel, comes to mankind's rescue and uses Frederick to carry out his master plan.

The book goes into the depths of despair and then into pure euphoria. Is this really a story of a mind out of control, or is this book prophetic of our future?

This book is inspiring and no other has been written to parallel it.

Dedications

I would like to dedicate this book to my late father, who also suffered from a mental malady. I would also like to dedicate this book to my GP Dr. B. Newmarch as well as the nurses who cared for me, and all sufferer's and carers worldwide.

I would like to say one big thank you to the Bristol branch of the Open University here in the UK for helping me to obtain my university qualification and for truly being open to all and not discriminating against me on health grounds. I am proud that somebody with my background was not too insignificant to study with you. Thank you.

Talmadge Emil Friedrich Rogalla, DipGerm (Open), CertNatSci(Open)

Chapter One

On many occasions I had visited my General Practitioner. I did not know or even begin to imagine what was wrong with me, but I knew something was definitely not right. I was very sceptical about seeing a psychiatrist, since it has always been my thought that a person had to be nuts to see one. However, the sheer psychological pain that I was going through was by far too much to cope with, so I took my doctors advice and allowed a psychiatrist to treat me.

My life seemed worthless. My mind raced around at ten thousand miles an hour, and I was incapable of distinguishing between fantasy and reality. My imagination was overpowering, and it had been ruling me for four solid years, during which time I lost contact with reality. My doctor told me that I was psychotic when I tried to convince him of my beliefs. I was rejected by a lot of people, becoming a victim of fate, blown about by the waves of adversity. The Department Of Social Security had not paid me for several months, and I was unable to pay my poor mother for my keep. Since she had a mortgage to pay, she almost lost the house and that could have made my whole family homeless. That severely worried me. On top of all this the council was threatening to take me to court. I would have to argue why I should not be sent to prison for the non-payment of the community charge. I did not fully understand my difficult predicament, and was too ill at the time to worry about the DSS or the council.

I was depressed, and I only wished something would happen so that I could be released from the agony. If only I could be released from the torment that life brought. Life was a burden as I was suffering intolerable mental anguish. I was leading a mere existence, and it was far too much for my sick and confused mind. I rarely ate and was thirty-four pounds underweight.

It was April 1991, and six years beforehand I had left my old School with good qualifications. I was renowned for being a brain box. I planned to go to college, and then on to university to become a scientist. Unfortunately for me, my ambition was dashed because I was struck with a mysterious illness. I was already taking medication and sleeping pills but nothing seemed to relieve me of the pain. I was suffering from all sorts of symptoms and two of those were anxiety and sleepless nights. My thoughts just raced around day and night.

I loved to listen to Radio 1 and my favourite program was “Our Tune” done by the DJ Simon Bates. It was usually a love story. I used to frequently phone the radio station to find out if the story was about me. I was in “La-la land”, and always thought that the stories were done for my benefit. I thought I had a long –lost lover .I even tried to get the contacts from Radio 1, which they unfortunately did not give me.

I had a crush on my tutor who taught me between September and November in 1985. She got married and had a boy. I got her address in 1988 and began to write her love letters, sometimes three times a day. However, I never got a reply. This worried my mother.

I also believed teachers who had taught me in the past belonged to a cavern of witches. I thought they had cast spells on me, so I read books about witchcraft to undo the spells. I often requested these at the library and got peculiar looks. I wrote to these teachers pleading that I wanted the spells removed, and if they didn't I would turn into a warlock.

I got addresses of past teachers from my headmaster of my secondary school.

I sent a lovely picture I drew to my old art teacher who worked at the Tate Gallery in London. She sent it back to me a year later and wrote "Keep up with the good work". I recall how she taught me about insane artists like Vincent van Gogh. It intrigued me as my father suffered from mental maladies and I wondered if he was artistic.

I also wrote to an old biology teacher who I once had a crush on. I wrote her love letters, but never got a reply. I even wrote a steamy letter to one of my kindergarten teachers.

As I was brought up to be a Jehovah's Witness, I studied with one of their leaders. He thought I was either suffering from demonic possession, or I was using illegal drugs. He often said a prayer to drive the demons away, and told me to read the bible. He said that when I heard voices I should call upon the name of Jehovah to make the devil shudder. Unfortunately, it did not help a blind bit.

My doctor informed me that I was suffering from a chemical imbalance of the brain, and that this was probably down to the genes I inherited from my father, who also suffered mentally. He referred me to a psychiatrist for the second time.

Previously I had been diagnosed as suffering from Manic depression, as I swung from mania to depression, and vice-versa. It helped for a while, but I did not like the regular two-week blood test that bruised my arm, so I stopped taking the pills. However, giving up the medication made things worse.

I told my brother that an angel had a divine plan for me, and my tales horrified him. I thought I had to save the world from nuclear destruction. Nazi's had infiltrated our defence and were forcing slaves in underground bases to build weapons of mass destruction. My mission was to make the world safer. I told him how there was a metal shield above an underground base, which was just a couple inches below the college foundation, and if you dug down far enough in the sports field you would come to it. Equipped with a trowel he dug a hole in the field, to the amazement of onlookers, but found nothing.

It was at the time of the gulf war that I had these thoughts. I even saw missiles coming out from the foundation of a multi-storey car park in a town nearby. There was a missile silo just by my bank's cash till.

Now I was allowed to write about the top secret mission called "Project Apollyon". The world will know that I am a Messiah who ended the cold war between the allies and the Soviets. I was chosen due to my loyal Christian faith, and used my influence on the military to benefit mankind. Now my mission was to complete my book sue the MOD, and become wealthy. It was the least compensation for all my hard work as I saved the government billions in revenue. In short I was a Son of God!

My mother did not know what the diagnosis would be but something was certain, I could not go on like this and suffer so horrendously. I thought that the MOD had drugged me in my past. This made me feel rather paranoid. I was totally obsessed with my past.

I walked up the road to the Tonevale hospital one April morning. It was drizzling with rain. My mother dropped me off at this Somerset hospital in the firm hope that they could help me.

I have had several jobs but I had often been sacked for absence, I could rarely work for a full week.

I looked back at my mother's car disappearing into the distance. My mother looked through the windscreen mirror at my sad figure and she only wished that somehow someone could help me. at one time I was such a happy go lucky confident person, career minded and successful, but my malady stole all these qualities and most of all, my happiness. The car's engine sound grew fainter as it disappeared around the corner, and I decided to hurry to the hospital as the rain was falling more heavily.

"Porche Ward," I thought gloomily as I stared at my appointment letter, "that is where I have to go."

Tonevale Hospital was a Victorian building with huge grounds -good for playing football. There were also workshops, where patients were kept amused for hours on end. The hospital had a pleasant and relaxed atmosphere.

Porche Ward was well arrowed and I could find it easily. I made my way through a hall along a corridor and up several flights of steps. I opened a huge door with a large round handle, and made my way into the Ward to the reception. The receptionist showed me to a small room in which a middle aged female psychiatrist sat. The receptionist introduced me. After the receptionist had left the room closing the door behind her, Dr Bolger, the psychiatrist, began to ask many questions. She wanted to know all the thoughts that had been going through my mind.

At first I hesitated and felt apprehensive, but then I went back way in the past and began to tell my story from the beginning. I had many interviews with Dr Bolger and I started telling her my story from way back in the past when I was just nine years old and met the angel Apollyon. I even had a copy of the story on paper, and showed it to her.

Some think that perhaps I was psychic, and that I was experiencing somebody else's experiences, and others believe I have engaged with one of my past lives. However, I believed this occurred to me in this life and that I was part of a secret experiment at the hands of the Ministry of Defence.

Chapter Two

They have a king ruling over them, who is the angel of the abyss. His name in Hebrew is Abaddon; in Greek the name is Apollyon (meaning the destroyer). The first horror is over, after this there are still two more horrors to come. (Revelation 9:11-12)

I ventured out into the garden one hot summer's day in the late nineteen seventies. In fact, it was so hot that a mirage could be seen in the distance. I actually owned my own plot of garden that my father had given me, which was now full of many beautiful flowers. I often helped my father water the flowerbeds in the garden during the summer season, as the summers were hot in West Germany.

I went out in the garden and laid myself on the concrete cover of the old well, and gazed up at the deep blue heavens. I closed my eyes momentarily, and then opened them again. I was wide-awake, but to my amazement I could see very unusual things going on in the sky. There were huge angels sitting on thrones, with crowns on their heads shining with splendour. There were male and female angels, and all were so very beautiful. A tiny baby angel, a cherub, was annoying his mother. She caught hold of him with her arms, and clouted him with one of her three huge sets of wings. They suddenly broke out in a cheerful chorus. Other angels played harps and flutes in accompaniment to a beautiful song. A choir of angels sang whilst an orchestra of angels played wonderfully sounding musical instruments and everything was tranquil and peaceful as I gazed up in sheer astonishment.

One of the angels descended from the sky with a carriage. The angels could not be seen by anybody except for me. The angel halted the carriage in the garden, and dismounted and walked towards me with a broad smile across his face.

"Hello Friedrich," he spoke gently, so as not to frighten me.

"What are you?" I replied, flabbergasted, and paused before continuing. "God perhaps?"

"No I am just one of God's angels." replied the angel with a twinkle in his eyes.

"Oh yeh?" I asked astonished. "What is your name?"

"My name is Apollyon," said the angel in amusement. "The king of the abyss."

"Why have you come to me?" I asked, hardly believing my eyes. "I don't want to end up in an abyss, do I?

"Young man, I want you to help me save the world from nuclear destruction."

"Me? But how?" I inquired with tremendous curiosity. "I am only a boy!"

"First come with me to my home," replied Apollo smiling at my curious questions.

Apollyon took me to the carriage by the hand, and lifted me into the seat. He got in himself, and the horse began to gallop and flap his wings, so that the carriage lifted off the ground, and up into the heavens. It was rather like being in a plane. The village became a tiny desolate spot on the landscape as we went higher into the vast blueness.

Apollo chuckled, as he watched me peer through the window. I had never been in a Royal Carriage before; especially one belonging to an angel. We rode higher and higher into the sky until we were in between the stars. The powerful horse galloped on and on pulling the carriage behind him.

In between the stars, I could see a gigantic city with huge gates leading to it. The gates provided a break in the walls around it.

"Is that where we are going?" I asked with great excitement.

"Yes, that is the place of kings and queens." Replied Apollyon.

"Why is the city so well fortified?"

"We want to keep the demons out don't we?"

We rode to the big gates, which had two powerful angels guarding it. The angels opened the gates and let the carriage through. We rode into the beautiful and magnificent city. The homes were carved out of all types of marble. On the corners were gargoyles and the streets were ruby red. The city glowed by itself, as there was no sunlight as there is on earth, although the city sky was of the purest blue.

Apollyon steered the carriage to a magnificent crystal palace. As he approached the gates to the drive they swung open automatically. We went a long distance up the drive when suddenly the carriage came to an abrupt halt. Out of the doors of the palace stepped a beautiful female angel.

"Oh hello dear, so you have brought the boy?" Said the female angel in delight.

"Yes indeed I have Persephone. Have you prepared the meal for our guest?"

"Yes, dear. I have prepared everything."

She stepped down to the carriage, took me into her arms and put her wings around me. We slowly made our way inside. She was amused at how I kept on looking into her beautiful eyes, and the way I explored her magnificent face. It was indescribable, as humans have hardly ever seen the faces of angels. She showed me the inside of the palace, and I became simply speechless and awe struck. Everything was so ornate. The palace was fit for a King but there was nothing on earth like it. Apollyon left the horse and carriage to the stable hands.

"This is an extremely beautiful palace." I said out loud, as I observed the many precious stones the floor was made of.

"Yes to earthling eyes it is so," she replied, "but now it is time for your meal, my love."

She put me down, and led me by the hand into a large dining room. It was like a great hall of mirrors with numerous chandeliers hanging down from the ceiling. She sat me down at the table. I leaned back in the beautiful green marble chair and marvelled. Persephone sat one side of me, and Apollyon sat the other side. The servant walked in and served the meal. I feasted my eyes on the many delicious things that were served. I felt really privileged. Much of the cuisine I had not ever seen before. It was amazing to the human eyes. It tasted so exquisite. We ate, and then delicious drink was served.

Apollyon explained political theories, such as Marxism to me. He showed that there were the workers, or the proletariat, on one side, and on the other there were the bourgeoisie, who were the capitalist. He explained to me that the world was divided between two basic powers; the communists and the capitalists. The capitalists want to make themselves richer, and hence they were victims of personal greed, but the communists want everybody to have a fair share. Both want world domination; hence the conflict between the western allies and the Union of Soviet Socialist Republics. Either was willing to destroy the world through nuclear weapons to gain world domination.

There was now an enormous underground network of tunnels, railways and motorways between underground cities owned by the west stretching right under Western Europe. There were also lots of underground nuclear missile bases. Weapons were manufactured underground to bring the USSR to its knees. People such as travellers, gypsies, criminals, outlaws, and the underprivileged, including communists, were set to work as slaves in labour camps underground, to manufacture arms for the western allies There was even an underground slave trade market between countries. Slave trains took slaves from one destination to another under heavy guard. If anybody disobeyed orders they were exterminated in special camps and incinerated. Many were often killed in front of a huge crowd to produce maximum control. The fear of being put to death caused blind obedience.

The soldiers who worked for the underground were very nationalistic and right wing. They saw the workers as expendable. The problem was that the western powers had fallen to Nazism, as they had once again infiltrated the western world's military. A huge brainwashing program was going on underground, and more and more soldiers were brainwashed to go and work in secrecy. The killing never stopped, and the slaves were too terrified to revolt against such evil rigid forces that belonged to Nazism. Everything was manufactured underground, including parts of nuclear driven satellites. The capitalist west is aware of this problem, but as far as the politicians are concerned they have tolerated this, as it was helping their political future. They were pleased that they could bargain and terrorise with the weapons produced underground by an illegal slave trade.

The injustice of the politicians penetrated all the way through every part of western society. Low public spending on things such as education, medicine, transport, housing, hospitals and high taxes are imposed to keep the arms race increasing with such ferocity, most people lived in poor housing and had lack of care due to the arms race, this trend had to be dropped before the man blew the world to smithereens.

The situation in Western Europe looked bleak indeed. Politicians were pursuing their own selfish goals, whilst democracy did not really exist. Democracy was a facade for politicians to gain votes. A lot of people suffered due to ignorance, but nobody really knew the miserable plight of the slaves who worked underground. They were rejected and long forgotten; always hoping for a messiah to take their troubles away from them; to give them salvation and freedom from the endless beatings that the NAZIS gave them. The underground was like a concentration camp. Lots of slaves died in appalling conditions. Efforts to escape were naturally futile.

Apollyon had intentions to change all this, through a boy he knew would be faithful and loyal to him. I was going to bring salvation to the slaves of the underground, before the NAZIS could use them to annihilate the USSR, and indeed the whole world through the manufacture of nuclear weapons. Apollyon revealed many plans, but for now I had learnt enough.

After the meal, Apollyon led me away from the table to a cabinet. The cabinet was full of silver and golden cups studded with precious shiny stones. He opened the cabinet, and took out a beautiful golden cup, which had a big red ruby on its side.

"Here Friedrich this is yours to communicate with us." said the angel giving me the cup.

"Thank you Apollyon but why do I need a cup?" came my very curious reply.

"You will need it in the future, to help the angels save your planet from nuclear destruction."

"Where do all these beautiful cups come from?"

"They come from the ancient tabernacle, where the Ark of the Covenant was in Moses' day."

Apollyon explained to me, that if someone were to drink from the cup it would replenish itself. If I were to look into the triangular ruby on the side, I would see the faces of angels and be able to talk to them, and receive divine inspiration. The time will come when I shall have to rely on the cup.

Apollyon led me to the carriage, and his wife kissed me good-bye. He lifted me on to the seat and, got in himself.

"God bless you, Friedrich!" cried Persephone after the carriage as it moved into the distance.

The horse galloped down the ruby red streets to the city gates. The guards opened them, and the carriage passed through. I held my cup and gazed out of the window, as Apollyon steered the horse in the direction of planet Earth.

Eventually the carriage came to a halt in Hoentrup, where I had started out. There was an old baking oven in the wall of the cellar which has been long disused, so I carefully put the cup inside and closed the cast iron door.

"My son, you will know the time when you need to rely on my help," said the angel. "Until then leave it where it is." Apollyon got on his carriage and turned towards me. "Be brave my little friend."

"Good-bye Apollo. Come back soon," I cried after the moving carriage in disbelief. Eventually, it disappeared into the vast blue sky.

Well that was a pleasant visit to heaven. I had to keep secret all that I had discussed with Apollyon at the dinner table in his palace. It was better that I forget about it until the time came to act. I went back to the concrete cover of the old well, and sunned myself in the golden sunshine of the high noon sun and fell asleep.

Chapter Three

I was fast asleep in my bedroom of the house, which my parents rented in the village of Hoentrup. The village was situated not far away from the town of Detmold, in what was then still known as West Germany. I slept fast until I could hear a rumbling sound coming from outside the house. I suddenly woke up and gazed into the shadows of my bedroom.

“What ‘s that?” I thought, as the sound frightened me.

The rumbling noise gradually grew louder, and the windows of the room began to resonate in sympathy to the mysterious sound.

“Is it an earthquake?” I thought with terror, as I anxiously got out of bed with the deepest curiosity.

Pulling up my pyjamas, I made my way across the bedroom, which was dimly lit by the street lamp outside. I carefully crept between the items on the floor to the window, which was already open. Now there was an absolute din outside. As I trained my eyes through the trees in the garden I observed a vehicle in the street, which had what seemed like a pole projecting out of the front.

“Good heavens!” I exclaimed, as I further observed the lights of other vehicles flashing down what was usually the poorly lit streets of the small village.

It was a warm summer's evening in the middle of July, and a gentle breeze blew through the window of my bedroom. It served a useful purpose, as it drove out all the musty air and left a sweet smelling atmosphere of a typical summer's night behind. The villagers at this time of night usually slept peacefully, but now the people in the neighbourhood were switching on their house lights and gazing out upon the sudden commotion that had woken them. The inhabitants were observing from behind their curtains and from the open doorways.

"Gordon Bennett!" I exclaimed out loud. "The Tommies have come at last."

It was usual at this time of year for the British army to arrive in Hoentrup on NATO exercises. The exercises were done every year in preparation should the Soviets decide to attack West Germany. The army barracks were just behind the Teutoburger Forest on the boundary of Detmold, only a few miles away from the village where I lived.

Lights flashed around the small village as the British Army moved in. Signalmen stood around with portable traffic lights and guided the vehicles. Tanks and jeeps roared down the main road, and the grating sound of the tank chains against the tarmac sent everything vibrating including the houses nearby. Soldiers stood around and gazed at maps under the street lamps, in an attempt to establish whether they had succeeded in arriving at the proper destination. A driver popped his head out of a tank and yawned.

I rested my elbows on the windowsill and gazed out at the commotion in the street below. To me it was like watching an invasion. Vehicles even drove on to the grass verges and anywhere else where there was room. The roads were chock-a-block, and military officers impatiently commanded their subs around them, in an attempt to create some form of organisation from the chaos that was occurring in the early hours of that particular morning. As the tents were slowly erected, the din died away, and gradually the invaded village became peaceful once again as the half moon gazed down upon it. The house lights went off again, and the villagers retired to their beds.

I stared at the motionless silhouettes of the tents and vehicles, but the only sign of life now was the intermittent glow of a cigarette that a soldier was smoking a short distance away, before he finally put it out and retired to his tent. I felt drowsy and wanted to go to sleep. After all the excitement of watching the army arrive in Hoentrup, I was very tired. I hugged myself as I retired and gently drifted of to sleep, as a friendly warm night's breeze ventilated my room.

The cockerel crowed as the first beams of light fell upon my face. The birds were chirping busily in the trees, as I yawned and opened my eyes. I got out of bed early, and crept to the window to observe the sunrise and meet the new day. I blinked in the morning sunlight, as my eyes had not yet got use to its brightness.

"Oh good, they are still here." I thought happily, as I gazed out of the window upon the army camp.

It was still early in the morning for there to be any life in the army camp. There was nobody to be seen, apart from a couple of soldiers who were on guard duty. There were always guards to guard the camp. I opened my bedroom door and quietly made my way down the stairs to the kitchen. I helped myself to a glass of orange juice from the fridge. I got up on the sofa, and gazed at the army camp as I sipped the juice.

There was a film of dew on the grass, which glittered in what was now brilliant orange sunlight. I watched the moisture on the grass turn into vapour as it angelically rose into the sky like a spirit freed from the earth.

"It's just wonderful." I thought happily, as I yawned for the second time that morning.

Suddenly I darted upstairs. I trod light-footedly so as not too wake my family. I came back downstairs with a bathroom robe. I put it on over my pyjamas and fastened the belt around my waist. Then I put my boots on. Unlocking the front door quietly, I made my way into the porch. Cautiously closing the door behind me I went into the garden. I stood in the sunshine on the garden path, and became hypnotised by the sparkling dew on the grass. The spider's webs were clearly to be seen, as they shone in the sunlight heavy with dew. I bent down and observed the tiny flowers, which were still closed as if they slept all night. Soon they would open in the warmth of the rising sun and show off their beautiful cups. I breathed in deeply and gazed at the rays of sunlight that bounced off the dew. I went into a trance, as the sparkles of light danced about in front of me like millions of dazzling diamonds.

"If only I could put one in my pocket and show my friends later." I thought as the mist coming from the dew rose around me. "I would show them to my form tutor too."

"Friedrich? Friedrich?" Shouted a man up the garden path.

I swung around as my father appeared of from afar.

"Good morning papa."

"Have you seen the vehicles? We have been invaded." Joked my father.

"Oh yes papa. I noticed them last night."

My father put an arm around my shoulders. Father and I stood on the garden path, bathing in the morning sunlight. I hugged myself, as it was still rather nippy. The sun had not yet warmed up the atmosphere. We gazed upon the army camp and chatted, after which we decided to go indoors for a typical German breakfast of percolated coffee and open sandwiches of sliced meat. Although it was my intention to stroll out that morning to get a closer look at the army camp, I never quite achieved my aim as I was so wrapped up in my admiration for the beauty of the dew on the grass that sparkled in the equally exquisite sunrise.

After breakfast my brother Roro and I made our way through the garden gate down to the bus stop. We were going to catch the bus to the primary school in Reelkirchen. Since we arrived before everybody else, we sat down on the bench and waited for our friends.

The bus stop was close to the army camp. The soldiers in the camp were getting quite busy now. They set up their equipment and stacked their rifles in a neat pile. Suddenly two soldiers appeared in the distance. They walked on the road leading to the bus stop. By the groceries they were carrying it was obvious that they had been to the local shop.

“Guten Tag kinder.” Came the greeting of one of the soldiers.

“A good morning to you sir.” I replied.

“I say, you can speak English.” replied the soldier in deep surprise, as I was still too young to be learning English at school. “Where did you learn to speak English?”

“My mother and father taught me.”

The soldier came closer and we got into a fully blown conversation. Roro was a bit apprehensive to begin with, but in the end he joined in as well. The soldiers came from England, and were training in West Germany as part of NATO exercises, which kept the communist war machine out of Western Europe. The most talkative of the pair was Peter Knor. He told me many things about England. My parents were planning to move to England sometime in the near future.

Uwe, my best friend, walked up the road to the bus stop and greeted me and sat next to me on the bench. The conversation between Peter and us went on.

Peter suddenly turned around, and shouted down the road. “Sergeant? Sergeant? This boy is English.”

A figure appeared a short distance away from behind a vehicle.

“What is the matter corporal?” Came the reply of a very attractive female official as she walked up to the bus stop.

“This boy was born in London.” replied Peter, lighting up a cigarette.

“Hello young man.” she said to me, and turned to Corporal Knor. “Well, don’t just stand there corporal, get back to your duty!”

She spoke to Peter in a tough voice, which made me tremble. Peter dismissed himself and his colleague followed suit.

“What is your name young man?” asked the sergeant gently.

“My name is Frederick in English but I prefer the German version which is Friedrich.” I replied, so surprised that she could so easily switch her tone of voice.

“As you by now know I am a sergeant,” she replied and went on further after a brief pause, “Sergeant Samantha Smith. You can call me Sergeant.”

She sat down next to me, and put one arm on the back of the bench behind my back. She sat in a very relaxed posture with crossed legs. She smiled at me, and gazed at me through her dark twinkling brown eyes. We conversed for quite a while, and I found myself immediately warming to her. Her straight long brown hair matched her beautiful twinkling dark eyes. That mysterious twinkle that danced in her pupils showed a latent sense of humour that blossomed as she spoke.

“I think Friedrich sounds much better than Frederick,” she said suddenly.

“I think Samantha is a very nice name.” I replied.

She lifted up a hand and pinched my cheek affectionately. Her eyes glowed with pleasure.

“You are a charming young man Friedrich,” she replied warming to me, “Where were you born?”

“I was born in Edmonton, London.”

“How long have you lived in Germany?”

“About seven years.” I replied as Uwe touched my arm.

“The bus is here!” cried my mystified friend for he could not understand the conversation, as he could not speak a word of English. “Come on Friedrich. Let’s go!”

I turned to the sergeant.

“I hope to see you again Sergeant Smith. I must catch my bus now.”

She gave me a bright smile that showed a beautiful set of white teeth.

“If you want to see the camp later on, ask one of the guards for me and I will show you.”

I grabbed her hand enthusiastically and shook it.

“Thank you Sergeant Smith. I would love to see the camp. “I replied beaming up at her.”

After wishing each other good-bye, I ran off to the bus and I had to hurry as everybody was waiting for me.

“Quickly young man!” said the impatient bus driver as I made my way down the passage between the seats.

“I have saved you a seat Friedrich,” shouted Uwe, as I made my up the gangway. “I wish I could speak English.”

I grinned and Anja, my neighbour and school friend, gave words of admiration. In fact, she was quite envious.

Uwe and I sat next to each other in all classes. We enjoyed making up secret poems about our headmaster, who was Mr Meier. We were notorious for getting into trouble through our mischievousness. In the Reelkirchen, primary school teachers could detain their pupils after school hours as a form of punishment. On the occasion where a pupil was detained, he could go home on a later bus that was always available.

Since Uwe and I made up silly poems about our headmaster, who was teaching us maths at the time, he ordered that we stay for an extra hour after school had finished. The poem was hilarious, and at one point the class laughed, to the embarrassment of Mr Meier. I, with my uncontrollable laughter, had disrupted the lesson for a whole five minutes.

The advantage of German schools was that one left early in the afternoon. In comparison to the long hours spent in English schools, the pupils in German schools attend only half a day.

After detention, my friend Uwe and I caught the bus home, and on our way we chatted about Mr Meier. We made jokes about him. I burst into fits of laughter, and Uwe could hardly control himself, to the annoyance of the students from Blomberg, who were also on the bus at the time. I went directly home, and mother served lunch.

Chapter Four

"Sergeant Smith said she would show me the camp." I said to my mother.

"If she is not too busy dear - why not?" replied my mother.

"Perhaps I ought to take the cap gun with me." I replied excitedly as, I finished my meal.

"Well dear, just don't get up to any mischief!"

I found my gun, and went down the path to the bottom of the garden. Outside the fence surrounding the garden was a road, and just at the corner was a checkpoint. Peter was on guard, but he did not observe me creeping around the black currant bushes the other side of the fence. A jet belonging to the Luftwaffe flew overhead, deafening the village, but soon the din died away as the jet flew further and further into the distance. I was going to play a prank on Peter with my cap gun.

I crawled on my belly through the long grass to the fence as quietly as possible. Peter had an automatic machine gun hanging from his shoulders. The soldier lit a cigarette, took a deep draw, and blew out a cloud of grey smoke. I lay in the long grass and loaded my cap gun.

“Wait until he hears this go off.” I thought with a grin, and pressed the trigger of the toy gun.

The cap exploded. Peter swung around so violently, that the cigarette fell out of his mouth. He pointed the machine gun in my direction.

“What the hell are you doing boy?” Bellowed the soldier. His face was as white as a ghost.

“Nein! Nein! Nicht schiessen!” I shouted with a fright.

In that moment, I had even forgotten to reply in English as I trembled with fear. The prank obviously backfired, and now looking at the situation with hindsight I wished I had not played such a dangerous trick on a fully armed soldier. Petrified, I got up out of the long grass that partially camouflaged me and made my way to the fence, whilst keeping my eyes fixed on Peter all the time. I held my cap gun out to Peter and he lowered his machine gun. Peter took the cap gun and realised that it was only a toy.

“What the hell do you think you are up to?” came Peter’s annoyed and embarrassed response. “Puh. . . toy guns. It should not be allowed!”

“But you have one and it is real.” I replied still shaking from the shock.

"That's different. I am a soldier and I need my gun to do my job!" he replied feeling rather hypercritical. "You gave me a bit of a shock."

It took a while for him to calm down. I felt really ashamed of myself.

"I was only having a bit of fun. "I replied feeling more relaxed now.

"If I had not known better you could have been shot!" replied the annoyed soldier giving me the cap gun back.

"I am really sorry." I replied wondering how I could change the subject. "Sergeant Smith said I could see the camp."

"Oh, so that is what you wanted."

Peter got out his packet of cigarettes from his breast pocket of his shirt. He opened the packet, pulled one out and returned the rest of the packet to the shirt pocket. He fumbled around in his trouser pocket, and pulled out a lighter. After lighting his cigarette, he took a deep draw, gazed at me for a moment, then blew out a puff of smoke and whistled down the road. A soldier appeared at the bottom of the road by the farm entrance where the headquarters of the army camp were.

"Can you tell Sergeant Smith that she is wanted?" shouted Peter.

The soldier put his thumb up, and disappeared out of sight. Peter turned to me.

“Well young man, never creep up on a soldier. It could be detrimental to your health.”

There was a moment’s silence.

“I won’t do it again.” I replied, feeling very guilty and I wondering what Sergeant Smith might say.

Peter and I conversed for a long while after which he lifted me over the fence. Then we sat down on the grass verge. The sun was high in the sky, and a haze could be seen in the distance as the heat distorted the view. Even the tar patches on the sun baked road melted and stuck to the bottom of pedestrians’ shoes.

Animals, such as lizards rushed about through the grass, or lay on stones and sunbathed, whilst the birds twittered in the trees above. I observed Peter taking off his shirt, and I followed suit.

“She won’t be much longer.” announced Peter. “You can’t rely on women, you know? They are always so long winded.”

I threw my head back and gazed into the deep blue sky, and grinned at Peter’s last comment. It was very much a thing my father would say about my mother. However, it was not very long before a woman who was familiar to me came walking up the road. I felt slightly nervous as I was wondering whether Peter would tell her of my mischievous prank. I crossed my fingers and hoped she would not be upset. The sergeant walked up smiling, and Peter went to greet her. He first saluted her, and then spoke to her in a low tone. I pulled my knees up to my chest and rested my arms on them. I was very unsure of the way the Sergeant might react to what she was being told by Peter. I hoped that nothing would be said to my father, as it would mean a beating for sure. Sergeant Smith giggled, and half a grin appeared on my frowning face.

“Oh my God.” I thought, as I rested my chin on my forearms. Sergeant Smith suddenly laughed and I sighed with relief. “Thank goodness she thinks it is funny!”

Sergeant Smith walked up to where I was sitting with an expression of sheer amusement written all over her face. Peter stood at her side, half annoyed that she did not take him a little more seriously.

“Hello Friedrich.” said the sergeant with a smile.

Her pupils sparkled like two diamonds in her dark tanned face. She wore a sleeveless green shirt because of the heat. She also wore camouflaged trousers and black boots, which were standard uniform.

“Hello Samantha. “I replied, beaming up at the woman.

“Sergeant Smith to you, young man.” bellowed Peter.

“Shut up, Peter. I have a voice of my own!” replied Sergeant Smith, who was annoyed with her corporal as he had a habit of butting in. “Back to your duty corporal!”

Peter walked back to his original position as he was still on guard duty. He was extremely annoyed now.

“You have given Peter the shock of his life with your toy gun.” she said with a helpless laugh.

I got up and handed her the cap gun.

“I told him that I was sorry.” I said grinning.

“So you wanted to play Tommies and Jerries.” Laughed the sergeant, and put an arm around my naked shoulders, giving the cap gun back to me. “You are a very mischievous boy, aren’t you?”

“I bet you he is a real little bugger if the truth was known!” shouted Peter from a short distance away, as he threw his cigarette on the ground and squashed it with the heel of his boot in disgust. But she just ignored his comment.

I put my shirt back on, and threw my cap gun over the fence into the garden. We walked past Peter, who stuck his tongue out at me. However, Corporal Knor made sure that Sergeant Smith did not see him.

“Would you like to see the camp then Friedrich?” asked the sergeant.

“Let’s do that.” I replied, full of excitement.

We strolled off down the road towards the army camp hand in hand. Most of the camp was situated on an old farm courtyard. Tents of all shapes and sizes were everywhere, and soldiers could be seen walking around. There was a particularly large tent where soldiers congregated at meal times or when they had to attend a meeting. The sergeant led me into the large tent. I gazed around and saw several men with crew cut hairstyles. They were also cleanly shaved. There was a large long table where cooks catered for the soldiers in the camp. The sergeant and I walked up to one of the cooks.

“I have a new recruit.” laughed Sergeant Smith. “Look Friedrich this is Mad Alf. He will serve you a drink directly.”

Mad Alf had flame red hair, pop eyes and a scar across his face. He certainly looked mad all right, but he also had a pleasant broad grin that made him look friendlier; or at least less frightening. I stared at Mad Alf as Sergeant Smith escorted me to the table.

"Do you like lemonade, son?" asked Mad Alf. I nodded speechlessly as the cook observed the expression of curiosity and fascination on my face "You are wondering about my scar aren't you?"

"Yeh. Where did you get it?" I asked. "Did you get it in a war?"

"Well I did not get it in a war that's for sure. It's not a war wound" replied Mad Alf, serving me a glass of lemonade. "Actually I fell through a chicken shed roof on my father's farm back in England, and I cut my cheek on the corrugated iron roof." There was a brief pause before he went on to say, "Where did you learn to speak English?"

"His parents are both bilingual." replied Sergeant Smith.

"Where was he born?" asked Mad Alf with sudden interest.

"I was born in Edmonton, London." I replied.

"Oh really. How old were you when you came to Germany?"

"I was one and a half."

"Oh well, you could not remember much of London then, could you?" said Mad Alf with a chuckle and gave me a glass of lemonade.

Sergeant Smith picked up a glass of orange juice and began to sip it. Mad Alf came up to me moments later and offered me English chocolate, which I gratefully accepted. The Sergeant sat down in a chair pulling me towards her and seated me on her lap. I leant gently against her chest and she put her arms around me.

"Once you have had your drink I will show you the rest of the camp," announced the sergeant.

"You are well looked after aren't you Friedrich?" said Mad Alf with a broad grin. "You're in good hands with our sergeant."

The sergeant loved children and she was quite attracted to the mischievous boy I was. She was not only good humoured and generous but also very affectionate which is something I yearned for. My father was a strict man. My brother and I were often beaten with a cane for our mischievousness. Like any other child I was drawn to affectionate grown ups. Since my father was brought up in Germany during the war he never readjusted to life in peacetime. So he expected his sons to be treated the way he was when he was a child through the war torn years. It was something that was totally incomprehensible to me.

"Friedrich, come with me," said Sergeant Smith, after we had finished our drinks. She caught hold of my hand. "Do you want to see the tanks?"

"Cur, yeh!" came my enthusiastic reply.

Sergeant Smith led me over the farmyard. As we turned a corner by a shed, vehicles came into view. There was a tank with its back doors wide open. It appeared that it was intended to carry troops, gauging by the benches along the inside of its walls. There were numerous instruments inside. The sergeant got in and sat on one of the benches.

"Don't you want to get in?" she asked pointing to the seat next to her.

"Cor , yeh !." I replied again in excitement.

I got in and sat next to the sergeant and gazed at the motionless dials. After a brief moment the sergeant led me to the driver's seat, where I observed the different gadgets. There were hundreds of them. It all seemed very technical to my mind, but I soon spotted the ignition switch.

"Can I start her up?" I asked.

"Hang on," she replied. "I must first check if she is out of gear."

After doing that she gave me a nod. She pressed the accelerator as I turned the ignition switch. The diesel engine fired up, and everything shook as the motor ticked over. The dials began to register. I jumped as she pressed the accelerator right down. The engine made an unbearably loud roaring noise. I was terrified. I thought the engine was going to blow up as it shook so violently. I covered my ears to shut out the din it made. The sergeant, seeing that I was a touch frightened, switched off the ignition, and to my relief the violent vibrations of the beast came to a halt. It was hot in the tank and our faces glowed with perspiration.

"Cor it isn't half noisy!" I said in astonishment as I looked up at the sergeant.

"Just imagine - soldiers spend hours in here driving along tarmac roads. That causes even more of a racket," she replied with amusement. "Let's get out of here and into the fresh air." Since the tank was stuffy and hot I was pleased to get out at last into the fresh air. A breeze was blowing outside and I felt the air cool my face. She closed the tank doors and turned to me. "Would you like to come with me for a drive?"

"Oh yes." I replied delighted at the fuss she was making over me.

She led me to the jeep and fastened me in the passenger's seat. She drew out a wallet from her pocket, out of which she pulled a pair of sunglasses. She put them on her nose before getting into the jeep herself. She switched on the ignition and off we went. She drove through the camp, out of the farmyard entrance, up the road past the local pub and up the track.

I lay back in the seat and enjoyed the cool wind blowing against my face and through my hair. We drove up a small track to the forest. A farmer on his tractor was on his way down. She drove onto the verge to let him pass. Deer could be seen in the distance, and a hare shot across the track as the jeep roared along.

The jeep soon arrived at the edge of the forest. To my surprise, the sergeant drove onto a smaller un-metalled track and along into the centre.

"Watch out!" shouted the sergeant.

I dodged a branch overhead and this dodging went on for a while. She was a wild driver but I loved every minute of it. Suddenly tents appeared around the next corner of the track. There must have been at least a dozen soldiers in the thick of the forest.

"Have you anything to report?" shouted the sergeant after stopping the engine.

"The insects drove me up the wall all night!" Came an annoyed reply.

I waited in the jeep as she spoke to her fellow soldiers. A soldier walked up to the jeep, pointed his rifle at me and imitated the sound of a bullet flying through the air. I slumped in my seat pretending to be shot.

The group of soldiers were cooking in the camp, while others took down their tents. The forest was full of wildlife. Beds of wild flowers grew in-between the trees, which were the habitats of the insects that annoyed the camping soldiers during the night as they slept. A wasp flew toward me, and I slapped it with such a force that it was hurled back through the air.

“Blasted insects!” I swore to myself and thought, “Why did God have to create such an annoying pest?”

The sergeant came along a few minutes later and got into the jeep. She carefully drove back through the forest to Hoentrup. She stopped at the bus stop and turned to me.

“Well that is it for today. I’m afraid I will be really busy now.” she said with a smile.

“OK sergeant. Thanks for everything. I really enjoyed the drive.”

“You’re welcome.” she replied, and wished me good-bye, then she drove down the road back to the army camp.

I was very pleased with my adventure, and I secretly looked forward to seeing her again. But for now I was more than satisfied.

It was still noon as I walked along the road back to my home. I almost tripped up in a pothole on the side of the road, and cussed to myself for not watching out where I was walking. It was not long before I was walking into the living room and greeting my mother.

“Did you see Sergeant Smith dear?”

“Yes mum. She is brilliant. She showed me the army camp. It was really exciting. . . . . . “

The conversation between mother and I went on and on as I explained my adventures with great excitement.

Chapter Five

Suddenly the doorbell rang.

“I’ll see who it is, mum.” I shouted as I ran into the hall to the front door.

I opened the front door and my eyes fell upon a scruffy boy who was my own age. Frank was my friend. He had freckles all over his face and his trousers and T - shirt were torn in places. Frank also lived in the small village of Hoentrup.

“I have something here with me.” whispered Frank quietly with a grin that was getting broader, as he quickly looked over his shoulder to see if anybody was watching. There was a mischievous twinkle in his eyes as he produced a box from his pocket. “Look what I have.”

“What?” I asked as Frank opened the box. “Cor ‚cigarettes!“

“Be quiet!” whispered my friend as he hastily put the cigarettes back into his pocket. “Are you coming out?”

“Who is that?” asked my mother as she walked up the hall, unaware that she had interrupted a very private conversation.

“Oh its only Frank mum. Can I go out?”

“Yes dear, if you want to.” replied my mother as she busily went back to her chores.

I hurried to get my shoes on. We decided to go to the other end of the village to smoke the cigarettes, which Frank had stolen from his mother. We walked past the army camp where Peter was on guard duty again. He let us through but he glared at us and stuck his tongue out at me. We took no notice of Peter and went on walking through the village. I told Frank about the prank I played on Peter and he giggled. Klaus, who was another friend of mine, waved as we went past. At the end of the village was a very old stone bridge over which we crossed before turning off sharply to the left and up an old farm track.

“I know where we can get some booze!” announced Frank with a big grin.

“Where?” I asked excitedly.

“There is a house at the end of this track before the gravel pit. There is a conservatory by the side of the house in which there are usually bottles of booze kept.” replied Frank.

Frank was the most mischievous out of all my friends. He had a reputation for being the most disruptive pupil at the Reelkirchen School. I had known Frank since kindergarten and we were very good friends. Frank had an older sister called

Anker and two younger brothers. His mother was of ill repute and she had an appalling reputation for beating her children.

“We must first check through the window if anybody is in.” said Frank climbing up the wall of the conservatory and peeping in. Nobody was in. “Come on Friedrich.“

“You can go ahead seeing as you done it before.” I replied in a whisper.

“O K. keep a look out.”

Frank pushed the door handle down and the door clicked open. He crept in. In the meantime I was getting anxious. If he got caught and the news got to my father I would most certainly be in for a severe beating. My father was a vicious man when he was in a temper, and my brother Roro and I received a beating many a time as punishment.

An old man came walking up the track, and I began to tremble with fear. The old man was quite some distance away, but my heart thumped inside my chest, as I quickly crept to the door of the conservatory.

“Frank? Frank?” I whispered.

“Yah?” Came a reply through the open doorway.

“Hurry! Somebody is coming.”

"I will be with you in a sec! Just hang on!"

I looked down the road. I saw the old man walking with a stick. He had a dog at his side. He was getting closer.

"Oh my God, Frank." I whispered in an anxious voice.

"What?"

"Just blasted hurry up." I swore.

"I'm coming." replied Frank, carrying a bottle, as he shot out of the doorway.

We ran as fast as our legs could carry us to the gravel pit.

"Oi?" Came a shout from the old man behind.

"Come and catch us granddad." shouted Frank, and he began to giggle.

We ran to the gravel pit, and then up the slope to the top where we had a marvellous view of the village. We were out of breath and flopped onto the ground where we waited until we got our breath back.

"What have you nicked?" I asked.

"A bottle of Schnapps."

"I hope the old man did not recognise us." I said still feeling anxious as I lay on the dry dead grass which was bleached brown from the summer sunshine.

"Don't worry! He is almost blind. Do you want a drink?" asked Frank.

"Oh Yeh. I will have a drop." I replied, unscrewing the cap and gulped the spirit. It burnt my throat. "Cor that is strong!" I gasped.

"Here have a cigarette." replied Frank, holding the open packet toward me and I took one.

Frank produced a box of matches and handed them to me. I took out a match and struck it against the side of the box and with the ignited match I lit my cigarette. I offered Frank a light and then threw the lit match over my shoulder. We felt grown up as we smoked our cigarettes and drank the Schnapps. A haze was seen in the distance as we talked and a breeze was blowing up the hill against our faces, which had a cooling affect which was rather refreshing. The wind suddenly changed direction and a cloud of smoke surrounded us.

"Fire! Fire!" yelled Frank as he sprang to his feet.

"Oh blow!" I cried. "Quick, put it out!"

"It must have been the match!" shouted Frank, stamping on the flames.

We began to stamp furiously on the flames but this action was futile, only ventilating the fire. It spread to other areas due to the roaring flames blown by the breeze.

"Let's scarper!" shouted Frank.

"We have no other choice. We are surrounded by fire." I shouted dropping the bottle.

We ran through a gap in the fire to a forest the other side of the hill above the gravel pit and hid. From our hiding places we gazed around in horror at the growing fire that we left behind. It was now out of control and making its way to the wheat field nearby.

"Oh no!" I cried with tears running down my face due to the smoke in my eyes. "What have we done?"

We waited amongst the trees and bushes for a while. The fire roared as it greedily engulfed the dry grass. There was a loud crackling noise, and an enormous cloud of smoke blew toward the village. People stopped in the streets below and gathered to observe the fire, which had by now caught the Wheatfield alight. The village policeman was also down below.

We better go now before the local police catch us." I said anxiously, as I was getting very frightened.

"Quick Friedrich!" replied Frank. "Follow me!"

On all fours we crept out of sight of the village people. Frank got up and ran along a rabbit path in the forest. I followed in hot pursuit. The path meandered around the trees and bushes but the general direction was down hill. The rabbit path led to a public footpath along which we ran as fast as we could. I suddenly saw something ahead, which made me grab Frank. We consequently fell over one another and went tumbling down the hill.

"What did you do that for?" shouted Frank in pain as he panted.

I put my hand over Frank's mouth and pointed ahead with my free hand. "See idiot! A police car?" I whispered out of breath.

"Blow! I hope they have not seen us." whispered Frank in reply as he held his painful arm.

"If we get caught the police will do us for arson." I whispered.

"Do you reckon?" asked Frank worriedly. "It was an accident after all."

“I don’t think they will accept that. We will get done for sure.” I replied close to tears. “I will get a beating from my dad.”

“My mother would beat me too.” replied Frank. The best thing we can do is get out of here!”

“I will crawl to the end of the path to the road. If it is clear we will have to go over the road, through the river to the hay barn over yonder.

“OK. Go on then.” replied Frank, rubbing the bruise on his arm.

I went ahead on my fours, and when I neared the road, I crawled on my belly making sure to stay out of sight and sound. Luckily the police car was empty I looked from side to side and ducked as a car came past. I looked up and everything was clear once more. I observed a while longer, and then waved to Frank the all-clear signal. Frank crept up to where I was.

“One moment.” said Frank, as he got out his matches and cigarettes and placed them in a plastic bag.

“I got an idea.” I replied, as I picked up a stone and threw it into the bag and tied a knot at the opening. “See, now you can throw it over the river.

“Good thinking brains.” replied Frank with a grin.

“Lets scarper!” I whispered. We ran across the road and down the embankment of the road and a little way further we came to the bank of the river. “Throw the bag Frank! “

He threw the bag, which landed smartly on the bank the other side of the river. We slipped without a splash into the river, which was refreshingly cool. A fish jumped, but I took no notice as I swam to the bank opposite. Frank followed, but choked on the water. I grabbed him and brought him to the reeds.

“Get your breath back and then we will carry on.”

“What do you think I am trying to do?” came an annoyed answer.

I grinned at my friend as we got out of the river. We lay on the bank for a moment to relax. I picked up the bag, undid the knot, and threw the stone out. I looked up the hill and watched the flames rising from the grass. Now there were vehicles to be seen on the Wheatfield, which was ablaze. The dry wheat, that was ready for harvesting, was highly inflammable. The hill was engulfed in flames and farmhands beat them frantically in a desperate attempt to stop them burning the wheat. The local fire brigade was on the scene too.

“What have we done Frank?” I asked in despair.

“Follow me,” replied Frank.

We walked along a disused overgrown farm track. We hid behind bushes as we went. When we got to the barn we laid amongst the bales with exhaustion. We peered at the hill with horror but there was nothing we could do. It frightened us. We lay amongst the bales and observed the dreadful thing that we had caused. The sky was full of blue smoke, which poured over the village, and now there were cars stopping on the road as drivers gazed upon the blazing hill. The police were everywhere, which frightened us even more.

The sky turned red as the sun sank behind the horizon, and the moon appeared as we maintained our positions amongst the bales. Soon after, the sky turned dark and the hillside glowed red from the ash that was still burning. The fire was now under control, but to what extent the Wheatfield was damaged was something we dared not even wonder. Soon all that could be seen were the silhouettes of the houses, trees and other buildings standing against the moonlit sky.

“Its time to go.” I said in a tired voice.

“I agree.” replied Frank yawning.

We got up, walked along the track past the farm and made our way onto the main road. We soon came to Frank’s home, and I wished my friend goodnight. I left the light that the street lamp cast onto the road, and walked in the shadows, as I did not want to be seen because it was rather late. There was a torch light in the distance and as I went further the light beam fell upon me. I was dismayed.

“What are you doing up at this time of night young man?” asked a man, whose voice was familiar to me.

“Hello Peter. I am on my way home.”

“You dirty stop out. You wait until I tell Sergeant Smith!” replied Peter, lighting a cigarette. “You should be in bed!”

The soldier and I conversed a while. Then I made my way home, and desperately tried to dodge the potholes at the side of the road. The moon lit most of my way home, and it was not long before I was inside. I only just got through the door when my father appeared. I despaired.

“Where the dickens have you been?” came a stern question.

“Oh, I was only out with Frank.” I replied very nervously, as my father was very quick tempered.

“Your mother has worried herself sick about you!” bellowed my father, and grabbed me by the flesh of the cheek with one hand, and with the other hand he hit me across the other cheek. “Get upstairs?”

I cried as I went up the stairs to my bedroom. I got undressed, put on my pyjamas and crawled between the sheets. Tears streamed down my face, as I was upset with my father. I was also fed up. The fire had ruined everything.

I cried myself to sleep and dreamt peacefully. There was not a sound to be heard in the village apart from people going home from the local pub and the occasional car coming past.

Chapter Six

I was enjoying my summer holiday now. I got out of bed, went downstairs and ate some breakfast. I gazed out of the window at the army camp. There was quite a lot of activity going on in and around the camp.

Frank came around that morning and asked me if I wanted to go with him to the local pub to buy cigarettes for his mother. I agreed and we made our way to the pub past the army camp.

"How much money have you got?" I asked.

"I have enough for one packet." replied Frank.

"Let me have the money, and I will show you a trick."

Frank gave me two marks, and I put the coin in the vending machine. I pulled the knob out half way, then reached into the vending machine with my other hand and brought out packets of cigarettes until the column was empty. Frank's eyes almost popped out of his head.

"Where did you learn that?" asked Frank in amazement.

"My brother taught me. You can only do it if you have small enough hands."

“I tell you what, I will give my mother her packet and we will keep the rest.” replied Frank, with a grin all over his face.

We walked back past the army camp. Frank held the cigarette packets in his arms. Frank was so thrilled at the trick, which I taught him that he thought of making a bit of money on it. Frank was fantasising on how wealthy we could become.

“Friedrich?” came a shout from behind. I turned around and saw a woman dressed in military uniform. “Come here Friedrich.”

“I am going to see Sergeant Smith Frank.”

“OK, but I will have to go home and give mum her cigarettes or she will have a fit.” replied Frank. “I’ll see you later.”

“Cheers until later.” I said walking up to the sergeant.

“Hello young man, look what I have here for you.”

I watched as she produced a bar of chocolate in a blue wrapper.

“Cor thanks.” I replied in delight. ”Are you busy Sergeant Smith?”

I opened the wrapper, broke off a piece of chocolate and put it into my mouth.

"No I am not busy at the moment. I have to examine some videos and that is about all. At the moment I am having a break."

Sergeant Smith put her hands on her hips and gazed into the field nearby at a pony licking its foal. The birds sang in the trees, and gradually under the observing eyes of Sergeant Smith and me, the ponies in the field came to the fence.

"Come on Sergeant. Let's stroke them." I said enthusiastically, with a mouth full of chocolate as I wandered across to the fence and patted the foal on the nose.

It was a sweet little pony. The sergeant bent over the fence and patted it on the neck.

"Isn't she gorgeous, Friedrich." she said with a smile. "I wish I could lie in the sun all day."

"Yeh. I love ponies and horses. I like animals in general. I have a few guinea pigs at home." There was a brief pause as I watched the sergeant pat the horse and spoke to it in a sweet high-pitched voice. "I wonder, sergeant, what films are you watching?"

"I am not watching any movies if that is what you are thinking." came a reply as she turned around to me. "In fact, I am sorting out some military films for my subs to watch."

“Can I come and watch them with you?” I asked, gazing into the sergeants dark twinkling eyes.

“Yes if you wish. Follow me.”

We left the ponies, and made our way through the camp, past the guards, and the sergeant led me into a viewing tent. There were many chairs there, all arranged in neat rows. It was really very much like a cinema, but instead of having a big screen at the front there was a large TV, which was attached to a video recorder. She switched on the TV and video recorder and inserted a cassette. The sergeant ushered me to one of the chairs on the front row and then sat down beside me. The film started to play.

“Sergeant?” came a shout from outside.

“Yes Corporal.” she replied recognising the voice.

“You are wanted immediately.”

“I will be back in a moment Friedrich. You can watch the film on your own.” she said rushing out of the tent.

I sat quietly and suddenly a picture of a missile appeared on the screen. The film was in English, although the presenter was American and the film was made in America. The film was about a new missile, which was invented in the USA.

The film showed how the missile, with its high tech computer, fixed itself onto vibrations from certain points on the landscape and used them for guidance. A plane or satellite marked vibrating targets. For example, the vibrating targets could be electricity pylons, telephone cables, motorways or buildings etc. The theory is that everything is made up of tiny units called atoms. Even human beings are made up of atoms. The atom is made up of electrons circling a positively charged core called the nucleus. The missile locks on to these vibrations and follows them. They have then applied these systems to remote controlled missiles.

Basically the same principle of the radio can be applied to the cruise missile. Dishes have been used for years to guide ballistic missiles. The only difference between the radio and the cruise missile is that it uses natural waves rather than those produced through dishes and antennas. Since about the 1940"s scientists have used the natural frequency of stars to gather information about our universe and basically the Ministry of Defence has used this science to develop its weapons. It leads to ethical debates about how man can use science and discoveries in positively helping society, or negatively to destroy it.

Spy planes are sent out to pick up and record the vibrations of certain points on the landscape. Then recordings are programmed into the Cruise computer and when it is launched it would follow the points recorded until it reached its final destination, which was usually a target, it had to destroy.

Another special feature of the Cruise missile is that it can recognise objects and hover and manoeuvre around them. It is very hard to destroy the Cruise with a heat-seeking missile as it is programmed to dodge an enemy missile. The Cruise is virtually unstoppable and it could be equipped with nuclear warheads. The Cruise missile is covered in a special paint that picks up waves and it does not use an external dish.

I was amazed at this piece of high tech. equipment. The videocassette ended and rewound itself. During the film I thought that somebody had walked in but I was not quite sure. The cassette was a reddish colour, which was unusual. Perhaps because it was top secret. The sergeant walked in shortly after the film ended.

"Sorry I was gone for so long," she said apologetically. "I have got something educational to show you."

She took out the reddish videotape, which she missed in her absence, and then inserted a video about NATO. She sat down beside me in the front row. The film explained the system of Western European Defence that kept the communists out. After the film was finished I wished the sergeant good-bye. I left the army camp and made my way around the village. I told various people about the films.

I went to Frank's home and met my friend. We went into the old shed at the back of the house and lit up two cigarettes. There were at least half a dozen packets of cigarettes there that we had stolen out of the vending machine. Frank went into the house and stole a bottle of his mother's wine, which we drank as we puffed on our cigarettes. Every so often, a car, or person came up the road, which or whom we could hear from the shed. That made us perk up our ears, and dash to the door to see if anybody was coming. If we were caught drinking or smoking, and the news went back to our parents, we would be skinned alive. I talked about the films I had seen to Frank, who was quite fascinated.

"I have something to show you, but only if you keep it a secret." said Frank suddenly.

"Yeh what?"

Frank went to the corner of the shed where a jumble of sacks were. He removed them and he picked up a rifle.

"I stole it from the army camp."

"Gordon Bennett!" You'll get killed if anybody finds out." I replied in astonishment. "It's totally illegal."

"Promise to keep it a secret!"

"I promise but I don't want anything to do with it."

Then Frank showed me the boxes of ammunition that he had accumulated. Frank got up to dangerous pranks. He often burgled houses but stealing rifles and ammunition of the MOD was a new thing.

"Why don't you take it back?"

"Because I want to keep it." there was a pause as he fiddled with the rifle. "So keep it a secret!"

I nodded and puffed on my cigarette. Neither Frank nor I inhaled the smoke, but the act of smoking made us feel like adults. I left Frank a couple of hours later and went to see my friend Klaus. Klaus was in his back garden with the air rifle that his father had bought him not so long ago. Roro was there too. They took it in turns to use the air rifle. I stood around eagerly until Klaus gave me a turn. He showed me the basic stance and made sure that my back was straight, as leaning backward whilst firing a rifle causes a great amount of inaccuracy. It's also painful on the back. He also taught me to squeeze the trigger instead of pulling it. After a few attempts I improved. Anja, Klaus' sister, came out of the house and greeted me.

“Hello Friedrich. Have you ever used a rifle before?”

“No I haven’t but it is good fun isn’t it?”

"I would not know as my brother never lets me have a go.”

“It’s not a thing for girls.” replied Klaus winking at Roro.

“You are a male chauvinist!” replied Anja in a little annoyed voice. “Come on Friedrich lets sit in the deck chairs and talk.”

We sat at the side of the house. We spoke about all sorts. Anja was a very attentive listener and the two of us were the best of friends.

It was late in the afternoon and the scent of the flowers flowed over the garden and wafted up our nostrils. We enjoyed the exotic scent. Birds sang a chorus high in the trees above. A field mouse scampered across the path, but fortunately Anja did not see it or else it would have frightened her. The lizards now disappeared behind the rocks. It began to cool as the sun sank behind the horizon. Suddenly shouts and screams were coming from around the corner.

“What on earth is going on?” I spoke.

"Oh its mother Prusser." replied Anja. "She is always arguing with her kids."

"What is it this time?"

"They probably stole something from their mother."

"Oh it must have been the bottle of wine that Frank stole earlier on." I replied.

We went to the front of the house, out of the garden gate and observed Mrs. Prusser chasing her children up and down the road with her cane. She was frantic. Frank's sister Anker had cane marks down the side of her legs, which were clearly visible as she was wearing a short skirt. Frank shouted abuse, which provoked his drunken mother even more.

"What have you done with my money?" screamed Mrs. Prusser at the top of her voice.

"You probably lost it you stupid fool!" shouted Frank from a short distance away.

"Just come here and say that!" screamed the frantic woman pointing to the ground in front of her with a finger.

"I am not that daft." shouted Frank in reply and I had to giggle.

"I am going to call the police." screamed Anker in anger.

The din died down after a while, and in the end everybody left the scene of hostility. It was so dark now that the street lamps came on. Anja wished me goodnight and went indoors. I was left standing in the street all on my own.

"Friedrich? Friedrich?" came a whisper from above.

I looked up and saw the nude white figure of Frank behind the bedroom window.

"Hello Frank. Are you all right?"

"I am locked in and I need to go for a pee." said Frank in a low tone, as he did not want his mother to hear him. Life was not easy for Frank as his father had died years ago and his mother turned her home into a house of ill repute after his death. She brought shame on all her family. "What shall I do?" he paused, "The door is locked!"

"Pee out of the window." I replied with a grin. Frank climbed on to the windowsill inside and opened the window further. Moments later down poured a stream of urine. I laughed and Frank giggled. "Well I must be going or my father will hit me for being too late home."

I walked home and on my way I met Peter.

“Hello young man.” he said in a depressed voice.

“Hello Peter. What’s up?”

“Somebody has stolen a rifle and a couple of rounds of ammunition to go with it from the camp.

“Oh dear.” I replied, blushing, but luckily Peter’s torchlight did not fall on my face.

“The trouble is I was on guard duty when it disappeared.” replied the soldier. “I am going to be in for a right cussing.”

“I am sure the rifle will turn up. I must be going home now.”

“Yeh I see you and stay out of mischief and if you find out who nicked the rifle tell me about it.”

“OK. Good night Peter.” I replied desperate to get away.

I went home and luckily my father was doing overtime at the factory where he was working. My mother made me something to eat before I retired.

Chapter Seven

The morning brought many peculiarities. Firstly, a well-spoken man knocked on the door after breakfast and told my mother that he was a friend of Sergeant Smith and that he wanted to speak to me. I met the man and accompanied him to the bench outside the house where we sat down. Mother went back in.

One could see up the path and observe the fruit trees with its ripening fruit. There was a silver birch in the garden. These trees were typical for Germany. The next-door neighbour's dog was chasing the cats into the woodshed, and a neighbour across the road was airing her feather bed out of the top window of her house. The sun shone brilliantly in the sky and the willow in the garden was a radiant yellow. Our neighbour Agnes cut the willow every autumn. It was a perfect day I thought, as I sat there sucking my ice-lolly.

"Well young man, I am a friend of Sergeant Smith." said the middle - aged man.

"How is she?"

"She is fine." replied the man and briefly halted. "I wonder could you explain the film you saw yesterday?"

"Oh yes. The one about the cruise missile was brilliant." I replied.

The man showed a great deal of interest in what I had to say. Then he offered me a lift to the army camp. I wanted to see the sergeant again. I got into the VW beetle belonging to this man and we drove up the road through Hoentrup. To my astonishment we did not go to the army camp but drove past the pub called the Alter Krug and up the way to the woods.

"Oh Sergeant Smith must be in the forest again." I thought still sucking my lolly. We then turned off and drove down a track into the middle of a field.

"Young man, don't worry I am not going to hurt you." said the man.

"Where is Sergeant Smith?" I asked in a frightened voice.

The man laughed and got out a case, which he opened and brought out a peculiar injection, which had many needles.

"Give me your arm. Don't worry I am trained to do this. Don't be afraid."

"But . . . . . . But . . . . . . What is going on?"

The man suddenly grabbed my arm and gave me the injection. I felt the needles prick my arm. I instantly felt very drowsy. The man picked up a CB type radio and asked for air assistance. I began to cry.

“Don’t worry Friedrich. We won’t hurt you. We will fly you to Tegel’s military airport in East Berlin. You know something the East has suspected for a long time and I think you will be a great help. We want to know more about the cruise missile.”

I was totally unaware that the video I had seen the other day was highly top secret. The film was never meant to be in the hands of the sergeant, but the MOD made a mistake. A spy informed the KGB that I had seen the film. The man told me everything and I began to sob.

I was feeling giddy. A helicopter suddenly appeared above the horizon. It came nearer and nearer and then landed. I was taken to the helicopter and strapped into the seat next to a blond woman. She put an arm around me to reassure me.

“My name is Heidi. We are not going to hurt you but we will ask you some questions.”

“I feel dizzy.” I replied feeling high and sleepy.

“What you have been given is Sodium Amytal which is usually given as a truth serum. It’s a hypnotic and a tranquilliser. You have also been given a benzodiazepine. It will make you feel nice and relaxed."

"What do you want to know?"

"Well Friedrich, what do you think of Sergeant Smith?"

"I like her very much. She is very kind to me." I replied and stopped crying.

She wiped my tears with a handkerchief.

"Well perhaps you will like me, too." replied Heidi smiling at me.

It was not long before the helicopter flew off up into the sky. The village became smaller and smaller the higher we went. We flew over houses, villages and towns. Cars seem to crawl along the motorways. We flew from Hoentrup to East Berlin where we landed.

I was taken from the helicopter to a laboratory at the airport in a Trabant with Heidi sitting next to me still with her arm around me.

"You are in East Berlin, Friedrich." said Heidi.

"Gosh. I hope you are going to take me home afterwards." I replied fearfully clutching Heidi's hand.

"You will be OK. Trust me. After we use the memoryometer on you I will take you back home again."

She led me from the Trabant into a building full of labs. There were doctors there that readily greeted me. They laid me on a bed and made me comfortable.

"Hello my name is Doctor Steinberg. I am going to be with you all the way through this." Said Dr. Steinberg with a smile. "We will give you another dose of Sodium Amytal and we will attach pads to your head and record the information on a memoryometer. The whole procedure is quite painless."

"Will Heidi be here?" I asked, as I needed reassurance.

Heidi Schulz, who was speaking to the lab assistant, quickly came forward and sat down on the bed taking my hand.

"Friedrich, I will be here for you all the way. Our country will be in debt to you for this." she said smiling. "The Russians will be very pleased."

"But the Russians are our enemies." I replied.

"They are your friends. Trust me. We will have a drink after this."

The doctor sedated me and put special electronic patches on my scalp. He switched on the memoryometer while the lab assistant adjusted the instruments.

"Now Friedrich relax and focus on the screen. All your thoughts will appear on it and we will record them on a video. Remember yesterday when you saw Sergeant Smith. Relax and remember."

I concentrated on yesterday when I saw the Sergeant and everything was revealed on the screen of the memory meter. Everything about the cruise missile was appearing on the screen.

The film I saw even contained the blue prints, which the Russians could use to make the missile. The film about NATO and the conversation with Frank were revealed. My thoughts were transferred to the memory meter, and then on to a video and everything was magically recorded. Doctor Steinberg laughed at the mischief that I got up to. The people in the lab laughed as they saw Frank peeing out of the window. Dr. Steinberg told me that the memory meter was a military secret but the British have a similar machine.

After the session with the memory meter the machine was switched off and the amused Dr Steinberg took the patches off my scalp.
"You are a very mischievous young man." said the doctor with a grin. "You have helped us a great deal. We are eternally grateful to you."

“Have you recovered yet, Friedrich?” asked Heidi.

“I think so, Heidi.”

I got up off the bed and stretched. The people in the lab shook my hand with gratitude. They said their good-byes and then Heidi led me into the canteen. We drank a cup of chocolate together. Heidi was absolutely delighted at the co-operation I had given, although in reality I had really no option. She bought me a bar of chocolate and an East German soldier came up and spoke to me and patted me on the head.

“The helicopter is being prepared for take off.” said Heidi. “Come on Friedrich, we must leave Tegel to take you home.”

Heidi Schulz took me by the hand and led me to the Trabant and the driver drove us to the helicopter. In minutes I was back in the seat, buckled up, and the helicopter hovered upwards and flew in the direction of West Germany. Over hills and valleys we went and I quite enjoyed the flight. We landed on the outskirts of Hoentrup. Heidi took me from the helicopter and wished me good-bye. She got back in and the pilot flew the helicopter upwards and off into the distance. I walked along the track back to the village and suddenly a group of soldiers pounced on me.

"Tell me you mischievous rascal. What were you doing in that East German military helicopter?" came a familiar and stern voice.

"Oh it's you Peter." I replied in surprise, as two soldiers grabbed my arms. "I went to East Berlin with Heidi Schulz."

Then I told Peter the whole story of what had happened. Peter was flabbergasted to say the least.

"You know what you did?" he shouted in dismay.

"What?" Came my anxious response.

"You have helped the Russians. I have to tell the sergeant about this. Get in the jeep!"

The two other soldiers, Peter and I got into the jeep and he drove us down to the army camp to the headquarters. He left the two soldiers guarding me. A minute later he came back with Sergeant Smith who had a very worried look upon her face.

"I did not know I was helping the Russians." I said with tears in my eyes.

"It's all right Friedrich." She replied. "But you have to tell me what has happened to you." I told the whole story to the amazed sergeant. "I can't believe the KGB could be so cruel to children. You poor boy. Go home now and I will see you tomorrow."

Peter turned around to me.

"And for goodness sake keep out of mischief!"

"Don't Peter. He has been through a terrible ordeal." replied the sergeant. "Good-bye Friedrich. I will see you tomorrow."

I walked home that afternoon very confused. It was an unfathomable situation to me. I went indoors and stayed in the rest of the day. I tried to tell my mother about the ordeal but she put it was down to a vivid daydream.

Chapter Eight

I was eating my breakfast as the doorbell rang.

“Its all right dear. I will see who it is.” said my mother.

I finished eating and a moment later my mother came through the doorway.

“Sergeant Smith is here to see you.”

“OK mum I will go and see her?”

I put on my shoes and the sergeant tied my laces. We walked out of the house to the front where the bench stood. The sergeant took a deep breath and then looked at me.

“My dear we are both in serious trouble. I wonder if you could help me?”

“I will do anything to help you sergeant?”

“Have you told any of the things that happened to you yesterday to your parents?”

“I tried telling my mother, but she thought I was imagining everything?”

“Well Friedrich, I want you to keep it all secret as you could be in danger!”

"It is very likely that we have a spy in the army." Replied the sergeant pausing, "anyway Friedrich I want you to keep everything top secret. You trust me don't you?"

"Yen Sergeant Smith."

"Well then Friedrich we must help each other. I am going to take you to the Teutoburger Army Camp. We will use our memory meter on you. We have to do this soon as the matter is urgent.

The Sergeant took me by the hand and led me up the garden path. We went through the garden gate and Peter was waiting for us in the jeep. The Sergeant and I got into the rear seats of the jeep, and Peter started up the engine and soon we were on our way to Detmold. We went through a number of small villages until we reached the Teutoburger Forest. We drove up to the guards and were let through. The camp was huge and we drove around for a while until we got to a building where the labs were. A man came out of the doors of the building wearing glasses. Peter stopped the jeep.

"Ah you have brought the young man. I am Doctor Simpson young man and I am here to assist you?"

After the introductions were made the Doctor led the sergeant and me into a lab and I was made comfortable on a bed. I was given an injection of truth serum Sodium Amytal and then I was attached to the memory meter.

"Now Friedrich I want you to focus on your trip to Tegel Airfield in Berlin." said Dr.Simpson.

Once again I had to go through all the procedures and the sergeant was dismayed when the blue prints of the cruise missile appeared on the screen. The Soviets could use this knowledge to make a super weapon. It was all one big mistake on behalf of the MOD sending the sergeant a highly top secret video instead of information about NATO. After falling in a deep trance, I began to think of the Angel Apollyon and my visit to the heavens. All this was videotaped, and the doctor and the rest of the personnel in the lab stared at the screen in disbelief. This is something that did not happen when I was in Tegel. I was given an injection, an antidote to bring me out of the trance.

"Friedrich?" said the sergeant.

"Yes sergeant?" I replied.

"Do you still have the cup that the angel gave you?"

"Yes, it's at home in the cellar."

"Do you realise who you are if the information coming from your subconscious is true?" she paused, "you may be a messiah chosen by the angels to help mankind bring peace?" she said pausing again. "You know a lot about the MOD and the underground network already. We must keep this entirely top secret. We believe you could help us in the cold war against the Soviets?"

"That is what Apollyon said." I replied.

"Come on Friedrich lets find the cup. My God isn't heaven is so beautiful?"

Another thing that was shown on the memory meter was the rifle and the ammunition that Frank stole from the army camp. Sergeant Smith ordered an officer to go down to Frank's house and pick up the stolen equipment before it falls into the hands of terrorists.

Corporal Knor drove the sergeant and me to Hoentrup No. 7 where I lived. We left the jeep and walked around the house to the cellar door. I opened it, and we walked into the musty smelling cellar. A window seated high in the thick walls let in some sunlight so that we could see where we were going. I walked up to the door of the oven in the wall and opened it. As soon as it was opened a bright light shone out from the cup.

"Wow isn't it beautiful?" exclaimed the Sergeant in awe.

"So you got the cup from the angel?" asked Corporal Knor.

I nodded and held the cup in front of my mouth and took a sip from the wine. My face immediately shone brilliant white. The sergeant and the corporal took a couple steps backward. I took another sip and I began to float off the ground. I smiled at the two of them who were utterly amazed. I looked into the ruby of the cup.

"Apollyon? Apollyon?" I said out loud.

"Hello my son." came a sound from the cup. "Your appointed time has come Friedrich, to work out man's salvation. From now on I will let you know my plans."

The sergeant and the corporal took another couple steps back through fright.

"What shall I do Apollyon?" I asked.

"Well Friedrich. I want you to let the sergeant take the cup back to the camp and store it in a safe place for you to use at a future date."

"I will be glad to do that your holiness?" replied Peter trembling.

I found a blanket in the cellar and wrapped up the cup and, as soon as I did that, the illumination in my face disappeared and I stopped floating. I passed the cup to the sergeant and she held it very carefully.

“We need to go back to the camp in the Teutoburger forest as we have not finished with you yet Friedrich.” said the sergeant.

She held my hand and we walked back to the jeep. The corporal conversed with the sergeant and told her that it would be best if they kept the cup a secret for now until they could decide what further action to take. They were both flabbergasted and speechless. The corporal drove back to the Teutoburger Forest camp.

“It’s obvious that the cup is Devine in nature.” said the sergeant to me.

“Yes sergeant.” I said briefly pausing. “Apollyon is a very kind angel. He is the King of the Abyss.”

The sergeant conversed a while with me about the cup and how I was going to help the British MOD. Everything had to be kept top secret as the cup in the wrong hands could mean possibly a war or something. The Soviets and the KGB must not find out about it.

The sergeant took me back to the lab. This time it was only the sergeant, corporal Knor and I present. Corporal Knor explained to me that they are going to have to erase everything about the cruise from my mind using medication discovered by the Nazis, as the knowledge is highly sensitive and could be used in the hands of the enemy. They gave me an injection and placed electric pads on my temples. I was made to remember everything about the cruise missile, and when I recalled it, I was given an electric shock that wiped out my memory of it. They did this for the information on the cruise that was inside my mind, as the information would be dangerous to the West if it were used by the Soviet Union.

After the information was erased from my mind I was driven back to Hoentrup. Then they gave me another injection to forget my experience with them that day. As I left the jeep and wished the sergeant and corporal Knor goodbye I made my way down the garden path to my house. I forgot everything that happened to me concerning the memoryometer and the method of erasing information from my mind. The jeep drove off back down the village to the camp and everything was peaceful once more and I was not a threat to the western defence any longer.

Roro and I decided to go down to the village centre to see what was going on. We walked past the army camp and were spotted by Anker. We walked on further until we got to the Prusser's house and to my surprise stones suddenly showered us. There was an angry Frank in the garden throwing stones at us.

“You traitor! You told them about my rifle.” shouted Frank.

“What is he talking about?” said Roro ducking away from the shower of stones.

“I don’t know. He had a rifle he nicked from the army camp and the soldiers must have found out that it was him.” I said, as I was unable to recall the meeting I had with the sergeant when I gave the game away through the memory meter, because I was treated with medication causing amnesia.

“It’s your own fault Frank!” shouted Roro.

Suddenly Anker appeared from around the corner on her bike with half a brick in her hand. I dodged her, but she threw it at Roro and it hit him on the ear. He screamed and fell to the ground.

“Serves you right Pucklesquash!” shouted Anker.

“Let’s have a look at your ear!” I said anxiously.

I looked at my brother’s ear, which was bleeding profusely.

“I will get them back for that!” I said shocked at what Frank’s sister did to my brother.

I picked up the half brick and ran up to the garden fence of Frank’s house. Frank was wildly scurrying around for more stones to throw. He had his back to me, but I waited until he turned and then with all my might I hurled the half brick at him.

"Have some of your own medicine!" I shouted.

The half brick hit Frank in the right eye and he let out one terrifying scream, which the whole village must have heard.

"Quick Roro let's run." I shouted to my brother.

We scampered up a road back to our house. Roro was holding his ear, as it was still painful.

"Cur you got him right in the eye." Said Roro grinning.

"Good shot wasn't it?"

"Yeh. I better let mum put a plaster on my ear."

We went in and mother attended to Roro's ear, which had only a minor cut. We did not tell her what happened and told her that Roro hit his head on a branch.

Chapter Nine

It was at last time for the soldiers in Hoentrup to return to the army barracks in the Teutoburger Forest. They packed up all their tents and equipment and left Hoentrup within a couple of hours. The children in the village watched the soldiers packing up and begged them for a piece of camouflaged material. Some were even given torches and Roro and I were given two tins of sweets.

My mother decided to move back to England from where she originated. Within the next couple of weeks the packing had to be done. My father was to stay in Germany and earn a living so that he could continue to support our family financially while we lived in England. He was an employee at a furniture factory and he put together pieces of furniture, but his job did not require much skill. My father was a German East Prussian and my mother was English. They met in Canada, years ago. They decided to live in England for a couple of years. Roro and I were born in London. We were born eleven months apart. I was born in my grandparent's house in Edmonton to where my family will be moving in the near future.

One sunny summer's day a jeep drove up to the front gate as I was playing in the garden. Sergeant Smith got out and walked down the garden path and greeted me.

“Hello Friedrich. Can you come with me please?”

“Yes sergeant but where are we going to.” I asked delighted to see the sergeant again.

“You are going to see a bit of the underground that Apollyon told you about.”

The sergeant led me to the jeep and gave me a pill and drink of water out of a bottle. Corporal Knor drove us to the army base in the Teutoburger Forest. The jeep went through the checkpoint and we drove right into the base. There was another checkpoint in the base, which we passed. We drove down a well-lit tunnel.

“Well Friedrich, you are going to see some disturbing scenes that we don’t agree with, but try and control yourself and don’t make an outcry.” Said the sergeant.

“Will we see slaves and missiles like Apollyon told me?” I asked.

“Yes, I think though the slaves will disturb you the most.” she replied.

“You mean they are beaten.”

“Yes they are treated very badly.”

We carried on through the tunnel and suddenly a railway station came into sight. It was the start of an underground city. On the platform of the railway station stood pathetic individuals in rags. I recognised these to be slaves right away. Guarding the slaves were soldiers with whips. Another soldier of a higher rank walked up on to the platform and two guards gave the Nazi salute. The slaves were loaded on to carriages without any seats. They would have to stand throughout the duration of the journey. The guards pushed the slaves into the carriage until they were squashed like sardines. It was quite disgusting as there were no toilet facilities. I watched the poor slaves and wondered how Apollyon was going to free them. They were pathetic looking individuals ,with the expression of fear written all over their faces. Deep inside my heart I wanted to help them at once if I could, but I realised that I had to be patient. This was a crime against humanity.

The corporal drove the jeep through the streets of the underground city. There were pubs, clubs, shops etc., for the soldiers of the underground. As we drove on further through the city we came to the ghetto where the slaves were kept. There were hundreds of tiny flats where the slaves and their families lived. Children were born to the slaves who, at an early age, helped in manufacturing weapons for the western allies. The children have never seen daylight, the moon, or the sun. The ghetto was very shabby and disease was rampant. Many slaves died due to the lack of medication.

We left and drove up a road leading out of the city. There were hardly any other vehicles in the tunnel. Corporal Knor drove fast for about a quarter of an hour when we suddenly arrived in a very large underground chamber. In this chamber were hundreds of state of the art missiles.

"These missiles are for biological, chemical and nuclear warfare." said the sergeant out loud as the corporal parked the jeep.

We got out of the car, and the corporal walked over to an engineer who was working in the missile chamber. The soldier saluted the corporal and they conversed. After a while the corporal turned around.

"Follow me." said Corporal Knor.

"Where are we going?" I asked.

"We are going to show you the missile silos." replied the sergeant.

We walked along a track that was used to transport the missiles and we came to a wall. There was an archway in the wall, which we walked under. The engineer spoke on an intercom and suddenly the roof above us opened. Great steel doors moved into the side of the missile silo and daylight could be seen way above us. At the same time the steel door at the entrance of the missile chamber through which the jeep came closed.

“In case of a nuclear war we are well protected down here. We have about a hundred silos.” said the soldier.

“What is above us?” I asked.

“There is rough land up there belonging to the MOD. Any person crossing this land is usually shot or taken as a slave.” replied the soldier. “It has to be kept top secret.”

The soldier ordered that the missile silo be closed again. The door immediately began to close. We returned to the jeep and I observed all the missiles standing up in the chamber ready to be used against the Soviet Union.

“Apollyon already told you that the western allies are preparing for a war against the Soviets hasn’t he?” asked the sergeant.

“Yes.” I replied. “We must stop them.”

“People have tried but not succeeded. We will do anything to help you Friedrich.”

Corporal Knor drove us back to the military base at the Teutoburger Forest, and once we were above ground we went into a specially prepared room where my cup was kept under lock and key.

"What are we going to do now?" I asked.

"We want you to ask Apollyon what our instructions are." replied Sergeant Smith.

Corporal Knor brought the cup to me and I took a sip of the wine. My eyes began to shine and a glow surrounded my body. I sat down in a chair.

"Apollyon? Apollyon? I asked gazing into the ruby of the cup. "Are you there?

Apollyon suddenly appeared in the ruby.

"Hello Friedrich. I want you to tell the sergeant the following. Find all the information on antiballistic missiles and lasers from the western allies, as well as that of the Soviets. Use the information from both powers. I will give the scientist the power of discovery to enable them to build a missile that will destroy all other missiles. With this information you are to build an inpenetratable shield for the Baltic states of Norway, Sweden, Finland and Denmark. When you sell the antiballistic put the money into more research, into building houses for the slaves, and the rest of the money into an account. This project shall be called Project Apollyon."

I did not need to tell the sergeant as she heard the conversation, and wrote everything down on paper.

"Is that all the instructions?" asked the sergeant.

"Yes that is all for the moment." replied Apollyon.

Corporal Knor took the cup from me and as soon as he done that the glow around me disappeared. He put it back in the safe and then we left the building. He locked the door and got back into the jeep. The sergeant and I followed him and got in the jeep. She gave me yet another pill and I drank that down with water. He drove me back to Hoentrup. I wished the sergeant and the corporal goodbye and went into my house. Due to the medication I could not recall the visit to the underground base.

My mother announced that we were going to go to England in a matter of days. She was already packing. Uncle Guenther and Aunt Edith came around to help my mother pack. It took a couple of days, but then suddenly one day we were ready to leave Hoentrup to find a new life in England. All my friends were assembled outside the house that I was going to leave behind. My father was going to live with an old friend of the family in Herrentrup, a village nearby, and still work in Germany to support our family when living in England.

"Well Uwe, my old friend we must say goodbye." I said with a watery smile.

"Friedrich," replied Uwe shaking my hand. "Take care. Write soon!"

Roro and I shook hands with Klaus, Michael, Anja, Sabine, Thomas and Frank. Frank had forgiven the grudge he had against Roro and me and brought us a bar of chocolate each. It was a sad event but we promised each other to keep in touch. It was summer of 1977 and my mother and my two brothers, Roro and Alex got into the car after saying goodbye to our neighbours. I was about nine and a half now and Alex was six years younger. The car drove into the distance and I waved like mad to my friends. Then the car disappeared around the corner.

We went by ship from the Hook of Holland to Dover. There was quite a powerful wind on deck and Roro and I went from deck to deck in the gale. We struggled to get up and down the stairs, but we thoroughly enjoyed the ferry crossing. It was a pleasant adventure for us. Soon we would be in Edmonton in London at our grandparents" house.

Chapter Ten

It was evening when we arrived in Edmonton. I vividly remember the red tarmac roads. As we drove up in front of Latymer Way Mum tooted the horn. The front door opened and two smiling people emerged. They opened the garden gate and rushed out to greet us. Mum was hugged and kissed by grandpa first of all and then by nana.

"Hello boys , come and say "hello" to your grandpa." said my grandfather delighted to see us. Grandpa kissed and hugged me and then Roro. Next my nana kissed me while grandpa got Alex out of the car. "Let's go in and have a cup of coffee, ducks."

We were all tired from our journey but I was very excited to be in London. Mum started crying. I don't know whether it was from exhaustion or because she was delighted to see her folks again. Anyway, it was a grand reunion.

We went into my grandparent's council house. The place smelt of furniture polish.

"Sit down and get the weight off your feet," said my granddad to mum. "It must have been a terrible long drive for you Wendy."

And so the conversation between Grandpa and mum went on, and my Nana butted in where she could.

“Are you hungry Frederick?” asked my Nana.

“Cor we are starving nana.” I replied.

Soon we had a cup of coffee and ginger biscuits to go with it. Nana made us some sandwiches and Roro and I had a feast. Then we went into the front room with Grandpa so that mum could stay and speak to nana in the kitchen.

“Do you lads want a mint?” asked my grandpa.

“Yes please.” said my brother and I together and my grandpa handed us a mint each.

“Tomorrow I will take you lads to the park. You can play on the swings and roundabouts.”

English television seemed strange to me. Everything was in a gentle tongue. I was already missing my friends. My grandpa talked a lot to us. He even sang songs.

“I am going to enjoy having you here”.

We watched TV for a while and then we went to bed. I slept on my own downstairs in the lounge. I had a sleeping bag and some sofa cushions to lie on. I was tired after my adventure and the thought of not seeing my friends again made me long to be back in Germany. In a way I was delighted to see my grandparents, but the idea of not seeing my friends again filled me with sadness. I was in a strange country and tears of longing to be back home filled my eyes. The pain of being divided from the country and people who I loved was deep in my heart. It was a lot to bear for my young mind.

Grandpa went to work next day and mum drove us over to our Uncle David's home. Then we met our cousins Joanne and Julie. I immediately took to Joanne and Roro took to Julie. We shared secrets and the girls took us over to the recreational grounds. We enjoyed our time together. They were roughly the same age as we were.

Over the six weeks that we stayed in London we met our cousins quite often. We formed an attachment to one another. After a few days in London Mum went to a place in Devon called Hemyock to look for a permanent place to live.

One morning a delivery van arrived and there was a knock on the door.

"That will be a surprise for you lads." announced my grandpa beaming at Roro and me as we all hurried to the door.

"Cor bicycles! ` I exclaimed looking at the two BSA Thunderbird racers.

All I ever had in Germany were faulty second hand bikes and I was delighted with the thought of having a new one. Roro and I were eager to ride them, but they still needed unpacking and setting up. Grandpa moved the bicycles into the outhouse and stripped off the wrapper."

`How much were they?" I asked my grandpa as they looked so expensive.

"Money in fair words." replied my grandpa chuckling.

He spent the next hour setting the bicycles up and oiling them. When he finished he turned to my brother and me.

"Do you lads want to come for a ride?" he asked, knowing the response.

"Oh yes grandpa, let's." I cried jubilantly.

My Nana came in with a concerned look on her face.

"What ever you two do, never let grandpa out of your sight. We don't want an accident with either of you!" she said like a mother hen with watery eyes.

"It shanty be repeated!" replied my grandpa reassuring my grandmother. "This day her children are safer because we made sure of it Rose!"

My Grandpa hugged my Nana. Roro and I looked mystified.

“What on earth do they mean?” I thought for a brief moment.” We were after all, experienced riders.”

“You’ll see.” replied Nana.

We followed Grandpa out of the garden and he got on his old fashioned bicycle and turned to us.

“Follow me six o’clock and stick to me like glue!” he said, and peddled slowly and we followed.

He was very proud of us and I felt really important cycling with Grandpa. We stuck right behind him in a queue and grandfather would peddle the speed we could keep up with. Nana waved from the door with a hanky. It seemed like my grandpa was on a mission. We followed him down Latymer Way and on to a street leading to a very busy road. It was the Cambridge road and I despaired. My grandfather must be mad.

“Grandpa, that road is dangerous!” shouted Roro.

“We are going to cross it!” yelled back my grandfather in defiance. If anything he speeded up.

“This is utter madness!” I shouted back but we were ignored.

Grandpa mounted the pavement a short distance before the main Cambridge Road. We followed. He cycled up to what seemed like an entrance to a tunnel. He jumped off his bike.

“Do you notice something?" he said to us as we came to a halt.

“Yeh, a tunnel.” replied Roro.

“Thank god the authorities had the wisdom to build a tunnel!” I replied, as I looked at the busy road and almost choked on the car fumes.

“Take a look!” he replied pointing at a sign.

Roro and I read the sign.

Notice: Latymer Parish Council

After a successful petition by Frederick H & Rose Beavan made to Edmonton Council it has been decided to put aside funds for a tunnel building project at this point after the accident of their daughter, who regrettably spent three days in a coma in Middlesex Hospital, after her collision with a lorry.

We are grateful for their determination to make this road a safer crossing point for many school children.

It has been further agreed by Latymer Parish Council supported by popular opinion, t o dedicate this tunnel to their daughter Wendy Beavan. By this lesson learnt we are trying to avoid this accident ever happening again.

Layer Parish Council

We were flabbergasted and grandfather told us about the campaign. They wrote a petition and hundreds of people signed it and it was even in the Edmonton Gazette. My grandfather was very proud to lead us through the tunnel to the golf course on the other side. He told us that this was a delightful day and thanked God that it was allowed to happen.

We did not fully appreciate what he meant at the time. Thinking in retrospect, if my mother had died neither Roro or I would have been around. It was an accomplishment for my grandparents to have the tunnel built. However, to see the children go through the tunnel of the person it was dedicated to after what was a near death accident is indeed a historic if not miraculous day. My grandpa wanted this day to happen. My grandpa was cheerful and when he met friends he told them that he went through the tunnel with Wendy's children. He would always say it with tears. We loved our ride. At first I wobbled a lot, but soon got use to it.

My mother was searching for a place for us to live. Her sister told her about the picturesque countryside village called Hemyock. My aunts were evacuated to Hemyock in the war. She found a couple of places and went to check them out.

One day the telephone rang and it was for me. Nana gave me the receiver.

“Hello Fred.” Said a familiar voice.

“Hi Samantha.” I replied. “Long time, no see?”

She knew where I would be living from Peter who had asked my mother.

“I need to see you," she announced. “It’s best if we don’t talk over the phone.”

We arranged to meet up in a couple of day’s time and she would come and visit my grandparents, who knew about my liaisons with Peter and Samantha.

As agreed she came to dinner and my grandparents told her of all the family members who did their duty during the World Wars. She was very impressed, and my grandparents even showed her photos. My grandparents took a shine to Samantha.

Samantha and I went walking in the park and she told me that she had a difficult job of convincing her superiors of the cup and that I was in some way spiritually appointed. She had to use all her powers of persuasion that she learnt when reading psychology at Oxford, before she joined the Officer School. They laughed at her and she made it so that that the least they would have, is an entertaining evening with nutty friends.

One thing that they found slightly curious, is that the cup was made from a metal unknown to man and that the ruby was an unknown mineral. This is why they still wanted to see me and did not pass it all off as a prank.

A meeting with military officials was scheduled at the Chatham Military base in a couple days. However, I had to comply and the situation was getting even more difficult, as the whole aspect of the underground bases and what ever I saw was to be kept secret. As I was a child and could blab away the secrets, a precautionary measure was taken to continue giving me medication. However, Samantha was going to spend some time with me so I could get to know her. This wasn't a problem as both my grandparents and my mother liked her.

It was agreed that in two days time Peter would drive her to collect me for the meeting and my cup would also be present for me to give a demonstration. Project Apollyon needed to be fully approved. Peter and Samantha wanted things to move ahead faster. This is why the meeting must be called.

While members of the Latymer household slept fast, there were three knocks on the lounge window. I slept in the lounge as there wasn't enough room in the bedroom. I opened a window slightly and put the thumbs up. I then left the lounge, went along the passageway and crept through the door in complete silence.

Samantha ushered me into the back of the jeep and hugged me. We drove a little distance to a quiet place and she handed me a pill and a bottle of water. Peter drove in the direction of Chatham military base as Samantha and I chatted.

Now that I had the pill I recalled the time I was at the Teutoburger Military base in Germany. I hated the scenes of the pathetically treated slaves. It was just like the concentration camps. This was working nicely. If all that Apollyon intended was to be put into action, the slaves will be registered as asylum seekers, and would first be placed above ground on military bases like those at Salisbury, which were very spacious and in the countryside.

The slaves have to have therapy and some may find it exceedingly difficult as they are born underground and have never seen the light of day. Even the open air at a military base is better than nothing.

Secret communities will be developed before the slaves are let out into the real world as asylum seekers on benefits. It was a huge project, and the first thing that had to happen was that the underground did not recruit anymore.

Samantha realised that I had a special appointment, which I did not fully appreciate. In a way I was a messiah. I asked her if it meant I was like Jesus. She replied that people like Moses, Buddha, Mohammed, Jesus, the apostles and many others were appointed. She tried to get hold of files about this kept on computers in the military bases. Apparently one file she wangled out of MI6 said that my experience with the angel is not uncommon. In fact most people believe in angels. Samantha always did.

Peter drove up to the gates and showed his pass. We drove to an internal check -point and he had to put his hand on an electronic pad, which scanned his palm prints and opened the gate.

We drove down a tunnel to a platform. Samantha pressed a button on the wall. I looked down a tunnel and watched a carriage come along on the mono -rail. I was amazed. Peter got into the front and we sat in the back. Peter closed the canopy and pressed a button on the electronic screen and we went off at a great speed. I enjoyed the ride as we shot through the tunnel past illuminated platforms to our destination.

We then got out and went up an elevator and along a corridor to room 101. Peter put his hand on the electronic pad which unlocked the armoured door. He opened it and a senior military official, who looked rather stern, met us.

“General!” saluted Samantha and Peter.

General Thomson saluted and frowned.

“It will do you and you career no good to come up with way out ideas!” blurted out the general. “I am a busy man and do not entertain such delusional babble!”

“Well, let us see if there is an element of truth in all this, or whether Frederick is ill. However, you know yourself that the cup is made from unknown elements.,” replied Samantha.

“I just hope you can justify your poppycock story Sergeant Smith, as your career is definitely on the line!” he replied and led us into a room of spectators.

There must have been at least a dozen military officials of various ranks in the room. Some were hauled in from MI6, which you seldom hear about. They were all here to scrutinize the sergeant. A psychiatrist was also present. We sat down in a row of three in front of a table which had my cup on it.

“So where do you find this cup, young man?” asked the general, picking up the cup and rolled it around in his palms.

“I got it from an angel.” I replied.

The general looked at the psychiatrist and she felt a bit awkward.

“Where did the angel get the cup?” asked the general not amused and there were a couple chuckles.

“He got it out of a glass cabinet.” I replied.

“And assuming I believe in angels, where is the glass cabinet?”

“It’s in his palace.” I replied.

“And where is this palace?” said the general beginning to feel that this was a tragic waste of time.

“It’s in heaven?”

“And how do you know he keeps it in heaven, in his palace, in a glass cabinet?”

There were more chuckles.

“Because I went with the angel to heaven”

`And don't tell me you caught the ten twenty bus to get there." he replied annoyed, as he felt he was taken for a fool. "Look young man, if you tell us where you got it from, you can leave and that will be the end of that. It will be freedom for you as obviously you are ill, and we don't really want to put poisons into you to protect secrets." he said sympathetically.

"I got it from angel Apollyon!" I replied getting annoyed.

`Balderdash!" replied the general. "Why did he give you such an expensive gift?"

"To communicate with him."

"I think this young man is seriously ill." said the psychiatrist after everybody had a good chuckle. "He is definitely psychotic!"

"I am not ill." I replied frustrated. "I'm telling you the truth!"

"And why would you want to communicate with an angel? And how do you communicate with the angel?" asked the general chuckling.

"I have been appointed to help make peace between the Allies and the Soviets." I replied and they laughed at me. "All I have to do is stare into the ruby and say Apollyon, Apollyon. Then he speaks to me."

The crowd roared with laughter, and one man started pulling faces, even the general began laughing and apologized to everybody for calling them to an unnecessary meeting. He mocked me and stared into the ruby.

"Apollyon? Apollyon?" he said laughing until tears came down his face. "What utter complete..."

Suddenly sparks flew out of the ruby. Apollyon was giving him an electric shock treatment. The lights flickered and went out. The general fell to the floor in spasms and let the cup fall. I stood up and walked over to the general and picked up my cup, which began to glow a fiery white. It started filling up and overflowed to the crowd's amazement. I took a sip and levitated above the floor.

"Apollyon? Apollyon?" I cried, and suddenly sparks flew from the cup and shot through the group of observers who were now petrified of the paranormal phenomenon.

"General Thomson, do not mock this young man!" came the booming voice of Apollyon.

"Good Grief! He even knows my name." cried the general cowering away.

The crowd huddled into the corner of the room.

"Listen to my servant. I have given him power. You will make anti weapons! This will save your planet!"

Suddenly I was lowered to the ground, and the brilliant light disappeared and the light flickered on. I put the cup back on the table. The general got back on his chair. There was a huge discussion that went on and the general agreed to make the three of us agents. He would get all anti weaponry together and also have the antiballistic made. It may cost a bomb, but now the whole crowd was convinced that I was chosen. In the end we left after the general saluted me and shook my hand. He agreed to all Apollyon requested.

We went our way back through the underground and I saw slaves in pathetic rags, clearing the roads. How dismal. They were under the watchful eye of the Nazis. Still, one day they will be freed and let loose. Samantha was going to keep me up to date with the progress on Project Apollyon.

It gave Samantha and Peter a real boost to work for the light instead of darkness. We all felt privileged, but also they have now got to do their research.

When we drove to Latymer Way Peter stopped the car around the corner. He shook my hand and Samantha hugged me and gave me the antidote. I made my way back and opened the lounge window which I undid earlier before leaving and climbed in. I got into my pyjamas and crawled into my sleeping bag. It was the early hours of the morning. I fell asleep.

Chapter Eleven

My mother found a bungalow that she wanted to buy. The bungalow was situated on the outskirts of Hemyock. We would go to school in Hemyock. It was a nice little quiet countryside village. The bungalow came with a quarter of an acre of land.

After a successful mortgage application, Fox's Park was bought and the furniture was delivered by lorry all the way from West Germany. After everything was in place, my mother drove us from Edmonton to our new dwelling place. I had a bedroom all to myself in the gable end of the house. I would have no problems going on secret night missions to military bases. I was delighted.

Hemyock was deserted on weekends but came alive on school days when the children from the primary school could be heard all over the village during break time and games classes. My mother had the telephone connected so that we could keep in touch with our grandparents and my father.

My mother sent my father photos of the place. He was delighted with the purchase. The picturesque countryside reminded him of the place he used to live at in East Prussia before the war.

The local Christian congregation in Wellington helped mother move in the furniture. They also invited the whole family to their Christian meetings. We went on the following Sunday and mum gave the overseer a thank you card for all the help the congregation gave. The members all beamed at my mother and welcomed her with great warmth.

I kept my promise to Samantha to keep all that I knew secret. Samantha and Peter thought it was a great privilege to help me, as both recognised my divine connection. However, I recognised them on their visits just like my family but I was not aware of going underground in any of the bases as the serum they used and the antidote caused amnesia of such events. This was to protect military secrets. Perhaps one day I will be given another serum to help me remember and I shall then swear the secrecy act, work with Apollyon to help the world become more peaceful.

Samantha and Peter visited us shortly after we moved in and came to tea. My mother was delighted with the company. Samantha told her about her Oxford days when she was reading psychology, before going to the military academy. I showed Samantha some of the pictures I had drawn. She was thrilled and said that I had a real gift. My mother told her how she won a scholarship and went to Latymer Grammar School and how she was invited to the Royal Academy of Arts. It was a meeting of minds.

Samantha was an incredibly warm person who got on well with people. My parents and my grandparents liked her. It is amazing to see soldiers in real life and not pictures of them at war. They are just normal people, but have to work to protect the interest of the country, and if need be defend it. I thought Samantha was very brave.

Roro and I attended the local primary school and it was a new experience for us. The emphasis is more on imagination then sitting and following rules as in German schools. Roro went into the fourth year and I went into the third. The fifth year is the last year before the pupils go on to secondary school. The headmaster greeted us one day.

"It's nice to have two fine Arians at this school." he joked.

"We are of Jewish decent." I replied.

The head master stuttered and stopped, then stuttered again and eventually turned in mid sentence, and apologized and withdrew the remark.

Samantha phoned me one evening and told me to come out and stand at the gate of Fox's Park for collection.
I went out of my window after the members of my family retired to their beds. I was ready for the next adventure, whatever life had in store for me. I looked up into the starry heavens and could make out the silhouettes of fruit bats against the moonlit

sky. I tip toed up the path and slowly made my way along our gravel drive.

“Hello Fred,” whispered Samantha hugging me.

Samantha gave me the serum. I swallowed the pill with a drink of water. I watched Peter fumble around for a lighter and suddenly there was light as he lit his cigarette. Samantha patted Peter on the shoulder; he started the engine and drove along the track as quietly as possible.

We went past the huge oaks and then the conker trees. The school children collected the chestnuts from the conker trees. They drilled holes through them and attached a string. Then they would play in pairs and see who could smash their opponent's conker by hitting them together.

I spoke to Samantha who suddenly produced an electronic pad.

“We have to take your palm prints Fred.” she announced, and rested my right hand on the scanner.

I watched a beam of light go up and down and taking a picture of my palm prints. Samantha pressed a button, and I could hear a dialler. She explained that now my palm prints were kept on the military security computer for me to gain access to the bases. She told me that they were sent electronically to the base by mobile telephone.

We drove through Hemyock village and up near to the Wellington Monument and took a right turn along the Blackdown Hills to Culmhead Military Base. Suddenly I saw a load of antennas.

“What are they for?” I asked curiously.

“Those are for spying on communications.” she replied.

“Is that where we are going?”

`Yes, this is Culmhead Base,” she replied. “Or otherwise known as Spy Post.”

Peter turned into the base and showed identification to the guard, who let us through. We came to a car park and Peter parked the jeep. We walked to another check -point and then to armoured doors. Peter, Samantha and I had to put our right hand on the electronic pad.

“How does the machine know that there are three of us?” I enquired.

“The infrared light counts the number of people.” replied Samantha pointing to the camera above the door.

The armoured doors opened and we went in. We walked along a corridor and went into a lift. Peter pressed level 11 and we started to go down. Then we went through a corridor to one of the doors marked Major Morris. We all had to put our palms on an electronic pad once again, as it was a restricted area. The door opened and we saw a middle aged man sitting at his desk reading documents. On his desk was my cup. The man looked up.

`Major." saluted Peter and Samantha simultaneously at the major , who saluted back.

"Hello Fred." said the major and I nodded. "I am Major Morris and have been appointed to you by General Thomson." he smiled. "You have already helped us a lot."

The major spoke a great length. He had researched all about the cups. He found that there were more cups like mine and he had a few specially prepared for me in two rooms.

He told me that there are about 144 cups altogether like the one I had. They have been used since the ancient tabernacle for prophets and seers to guide people. The cups signify a vow, just like the cup of Christ meant a vow between him and the apostles. Just like Jesus spoke of his cup he made with God.

However, there are two types of cups. There are also the cup of demons. There are in total 666 cups of demons. They that drink from these cups will receive eternal damnation. They shall be obliterated forever.

- Major Morris told me about how he found 12 cups like mine and 6 cups of the demons. Both types of cupbearers are working for the MOD. He told me that I must stay faithful to Apollyon even under test. Then I shall inherit life as a spirit creature and have immortality.

Several of the cups had been experimented with. The metals were copied to make new types of planes with a quantum engine that pulsates light. It replenishes itself from the universal ether, or energy.

The MOD was using information from the cups to try and find the solution to world peace. I was what they have been waiting for. However, there exists a struggle between good and evil and the evil side will try and stop me. I had to prove faithful under test.

The major pressed a switch and a doorway appeared in the side of the wall. He walked us through to a room of twelve beautiful studded cups. They were so ornate. I drank from my cup and went brilliant white. It blinded the other three. The energy was so intense. The major was not surprised as he had seen all this before. I put the cup down and looked at all the other cups.

“They belong to your spiritual brethren.” he said to me.

“Aren’t they beautiful.” smiled Samantha.

“Are you ready for you test Fred?” asked the major.

“What is the test?” I asked.

“I shall show you.”

“I don’t think he ought to, just yet!” replied Peter.

“Nonsense, he is more than prepared!” replied the major. He led me to another room and unlocked the door. “You must follow you heart.”

I opened the door and slowly walked in the dark room, which smelt musty. Suddenly, as if switched on by light, six dull silver cups turned shiny gold and their black stones turned to ruby.

“Very deceptive!” I thought.

I picked one up and I could see a face of a woman in the ruby.

“Drink Frederick, my dear boy. Drink your fill and know good and bad!”

The cup was alluring as I could here soft music like the harps of angels. Major Morris had made a mistake. This cup too belonged to the angels. Gleefully I looked into the ruby and lifted it near my lips.

"Apollyon? Apollyon?" I cried and the cup filled with smoke that wafted all over the place, and smelt like burnt flesh. It turned a dull silver and I dropped it in horror. I ran from the room and locked the door.

"Did you drink from the cups?" asked the Major.

"Certainly not!" I replied. "They are full of filth." I paused "Very deceptive!"

"You have past your test." beamed the major, and Samantha and Peter cheered.

I drank from Apollyon cup and I gave instruction to the major about Project Apollyon, which he noted down. He then promised to get things in order. He was delighted to say the least, and wanted to co-operate fully.

Samantha and Peter took me home again and gave me the antidote. I rested a couple weeks before my next Rendezvous.

Chapter Twelve

I crept out of my window and followed the path and then we drove out of Fox's Park. Samantha gave me the serum as usual. I swallowed the pill with water, and suddenly all the knowledge of all the secret missions to the underground installations came back into my memory.

"Where are we going tonight?" I asked.

"We are going to the Manor Camp in Norton Fitzwarren." she replied as Peter lit his usual cigarette.

"What are we going to do there?"

"We are going to introduce you to a very old part of the underground."

We went down Wellington Hill in the direction of the Manor Camp in Norton Fitzwarren.

I could suddenly see rows of barbed wire fences. I realised why we had to pay so much tax. It all went into these multibillion pound bases. It must cost a bomb!

Peter showed the guard his identification and we were let through. He drove into the camp and went to another checkpoint, where we all had to scan in our palm prints. The computer opened the gate and we drove down a lit tunnel to the base under Taunton.

We came to the underground city. I observed the slaves working on ballistic missiles under the careful watch of Nazi guards. I pitied the slaves, who were mostly children. The life expectancy was low. They coughed, looked gaunt and wore rags.

"When will they be set free Samantha?" I asked curiously.

"When Project Apollyon is up and running." she replied." We are presently making the antiballistic called PEACE. They even have lasers attached to them."

"So freedom for them is a step closer?"

"Yes." She replied smiling. "It's all down to you, you know?"

Peter halted the car, and we watched the slaves work in various workshops. It was a dreadful sight. If it wasn't for Apollyon the slaves would never taste freedom.

The slaves were assembling various missiles with different warheads. They worked with great intensity. Peter drove to the underground hospital. He stopped the car and we went in through the double doors. There were rows and rows of cots full of babies.

"Where did all these babies come from?" I asked flabbergasted.

"They are born to the underground slaves." replied Samantha, touching the toes of one of the little babies and smiled. "A pregnant slave is given better treatment and food. They need these new comers to build weaponry."

I was utterly horrified. How could anybody be so cruel? It was like a human factory. I was baffled to say the least.

Peter took us back to the jeep and we drove through a tunnel that ended up with a dead end.

"Now we are going to show you part of the old underground." announced Samantha walking up to a door. "We have to walk our way there."

She pressed a number on a key pad, and the door opened upwards revealing a large black mouth. Peter gave us a torch each, and we walked up the tunnel. There were drips of water coming from the ceiling. We dodged puddles. Samantha walked up to a box on the side of the tunnel and opened it. She moved the lever down and lights came on in the passage. We walked up further and came to a junction. We turned left and came to a door. Peter opened the door, which wasn't locked and we ended up in a cellar with a wine bar.

"Where are we?" I asked.

"At the Freemason's Lodge." replied Peter.

We made our way upstairs and entered the lodge. It was like a temple with a chequered black and white tiled floor and pillars going from the floor to the ceiling.

"Why have you brought me here?" I asked.

"This is where people worship the lord of darkness." Replied Samantha. "Followers of the wild beast of Babylon."

I looked around and saw books which contained mysterious rituals to Egyptian gods. The temple had a weird uninviting atmosphere.

"People here use the cup of demons," replied Peter. "And you are not one of them." he said smiling.

There were posh chairs facing into the middle from the North, East, South and West. What a strange place.

"There are quite a few masons amongst the high rankers in the military.." said Samantha looking down at me.

We left the hall, made our way back through the cellar and into the tunnel. Peter closed the door; we walked back to the junction and walked along another tunnel until we came to yet another door.

"Be ever so quiet." whispered Peter, opening the door. "This leads to the dungeon of the police station."

I looked around and saw about half a dozen cells, which were painted black. The doors were made from heavy wrought iron. There was a torture chamber with various devices too. I saw a flight of steps and pointed my torch upwards.

"That leads to the used part of the police station." said Samantha.

We heard a noise from above and decided to leave. We hurried through the door and closed it behind us. We walked around a corner and went some way and came to another door. Peter opened the door and it came to the underground part of the hospital.

I saw a number of body parts pickled in large jars. This was extremely eerie. I wanted to leave right away.

"The steps lead to the Mortuary." grinned Peter.

Samantha hugged her arms and I shivered.

“I don’t like it here.” I replied and we went back out and closed the door behind us,

Suddenly there was a banging noise.

“Who goes there? Friend or Foe?” shouted somebody.

“Is that a ghost?” I cried and hurried as fast as I could.

We soon came to the light switch and Peter moved the lever upwards until the lights went off.

“Who goes there?” came a cry.

“It’s a ghost!” I cried terrified.

“Come on Frederick.” said Samantha pulling me along.

We got to the door and Peter put in the numbers, the door opened and I leapt through into the well lit tunnel. We got into the jeep and sped off.

“Was that a ghost?” I asked.

“No, a night watchman.” replied Samantha. “He also sounded like a mason.”

“Not a ghost then?”

“No, not a ghost.” replied Samantha reassuring me.

Chapter Thirteen

It came about that the big day arrived when the PEACE missile would be tried out. We made arrangements to go to the manor camp again. If the missile worked the slaves would go free.

Peter was in the driver's seat of the jeep. I was given the serum and all the other times when I was drugged came back to my mind. However, I could not remember any of my secret meetings with Samantha after the antidote was given. It was like having a mental block.

"Come on. Get in the back with me." she said whispering and I obeyed.

Peter drove us through the streets of Wellington and we ended up at Manor Camp. Samantha explained to me that the MOD collected all the antiballistic secrets from the USSR and the USA for research. A new antiballistic missile was made with a similar device like the cruise computer.

Today there existed a Baltic shield between the Baltic countries and the USSR. Tonight it was going to be tested. The Baltic countries were given this high tech device to prevent nuclear missiles from entering their country. The antiballistic was small, undetectable, and nimble and could fly greater distances than any before.

After trials the Baltic States challenged the USSR to send twenty unarmed nuclear missiles betting that they could shoot them down over Soviet soil with their high tech antiballistic. The USSR scoffed at this, but nevertheless they agreed to the experiment.

We went through a checkpoint and then drove through a tunnel to an underground base. We went to a top security unit where Samantha had to use an electronic card to open the heavy armoured steel doors. We went in and there were many people inside a hall sitting behind computers and monitors. At the front of the hall was a giant electronic map.

"Hello Sergeant Smith." greeted a commander.

"Hello commander. I have brought the boy."

"Well young man, we are going to test out the new high tech PEACE missile produced here in England." said the Commander. "You can rely on the British for new inventions."

He showed us to our seats. There was a great deal of communication going on. I was witnessing project Apollyon that was a top-secret operation. The missile-testing site was to be held over an unpopulated area east of the Baltic.

"Do you think this is going to work commander?" asked Samantha.

"I hope so." was the brief reply.

At 2:00 am, 30th June 1978 the experiment began.

"All stations to Defcon 4" said the commander into his microphone.

The Soviet bases were preparing their missiles to be fired into the Baltic States, so it was only natural to prepare for nuclear war in case something went wrong. More Soviet Silos were opened.

"Move to Defcon 3, came the commander's voice. "Alert Baltic stations. Prepare PEACE."

The computers were flashing from one screen to the next and the personnel became very active. In case the Soviets decided to play foul and send an arsenal of nuclear tipped missiles the Western Command had to prepare for retaliation. All Soviet missile bases were opened which was tracked by satellite. The station alarms were actuated.

"Move to Defcon 2."

The missiles were prepared for launching. The launch commenced and the electronic world map was tracking them as they shot into the Soviet skies.

“Move to Defcon 1 and stand by for counter attack,” bellowed the commander as perspiration dripped down his face.

There was sheer silence all around the station. The whole West was stood on red alert as the twenty Soviet missiles approached the Baltic States. Fortunately, the Soviets were playing fair and only sent twenty missiles. Otherwise it would signify nuclear war. The commander held his breath but to everybody’s relief the missiles disappeared off the screen. The personnel stood up and gradually they all began to cheer and clap. All the missiles disappeared from the screen having failed to arrive at their intended destination. Suddenly the personnel on the command station broke out in rapturous cheering. The commander turned to me.

“Yes…Yes……Yes…Yes!” he said hugging me. “This could signify the end of the Cold War.”

“Well done Friedrich.” cried Samantha as she hugged the commander and me.

“For goodness sake, move to Defcon 4 and switch off that alarm.” shouted the ecstatic commander. “Congratulations young man.” “This is just incredible!”

Samantha took me to a bar in the underground city. She bought me a drink and we spoke. She told me that the new high tech antiballistic missile could spell the end of the cold war.

Soon the slaves on the underground could be let go as this meant that the West was not so desperate for armaments any longer. The Baltic States bought up the antiballistic for experimental purposes and the money was deposited in a Swiss bank under the name of Apollyon. This Swiss bank now took over the funds of Sweden, Norway, Denmark and Finland. The Apollyon account was there for research into antiballistic and for housing the slaves. No money would be lent for or spent on weapons. The USSR, the USA and all western countries bought the antiballistic. The Apollyon account grew by the second. Soon the Bank of America, the Deutsche Bundesbank and banks of the USSR were taken over by the Swiss bank with the Apollyon account. This meant less and less money for weapons. At last peace has been reached and the slaves would be rehoused.

Chapter Fourteen

I was feeling unwell. Mother thought that I should see a doctor. About two years have passed since we moved to England. My visits from Peter and Samantha became more infrequent. I started the Secondary School in September 1980 and I was not doing so well at exams. I felt mentally sick. I felt exhausted and run down. I kept having hallucinations of angels, but I kept them to myself.

Samantha explained to me that quite a lot of the slaves were released to bases such as the one at Salisbury Plain. The money from the PEACE Missile was used to build the slaves homes, feed them and treat them. Even a hospital was built for them.

However, there were pockets of resistance; the main one being under the Salisbury Base to where the Slaves were transported. The Nazi's did not want to lose control of their authority in the underground bases. They refused exit counselling designed by Samantha and colleagues.

I had visited the military base at Salisbury Plain and about a thousand slaves were housed there then. The figure was growing by the day. General Thomson got permission for all of this. It was planned that the slaves would gradually be integrated into society.

I was really delighted that the slaves were released. I saw a film of the new PEACE missile, which had made such an impact on our MOD. The Apollyon account grew by the second. There was plenty of money for the slaves, to house them, to feed them, to give them medical care and to pay them benefits. Now variants of the PEACE missile were made. Some could knock out tanks, radar stations, satellites, submarines and also ships. Its highpowered laser could shoot objects from the sky. The research was highly successful and the money was used for peaceful purposes.

I was often extremely sick when I went on the underground with Samantha. They realised that the drugs they gave to me had this affect and were now concerned with the long term side effects. However, my work was not yet complete. I had to do a tiny bit more and Peter and Samantha encouraged me.

I was faithful to Apollyon and I wanted to help build a peaceful world. I wanted to see every slave released and given dignity and respect. The Nazi's were drinking in the last chance saloon and knew it. We won every battle but now we had to win the war. It was D-Day.

On this particular day in the high summer I was picking dandelions for my rabbit along the hedges of our lane. I was just outside of Fox's Park. I had a rabbit that I called Bugsy. I adored my temperamental bunny.

Suddenly a jeep arrived and came to a stand still.

“Frederick, it's D-Day.” cried Samantha.

I recognised the two, put the dandelions on the verge and got in the back of the jeep with Samantha.

“Another mission to God knows where.” I said swallowing the serum with a grin.

“Frederick, this is the final moment...its D-Day!” replied Samantha. “Soon you will be released from the MOD.”

“How can I help?” I asked.

“We are experiencing resistance from the Nazi's under Salisbury Base.” she replied.” They want to detain the slaves. We are going to rely on you and the cup. This is an order from General Thomson. The people of darkness are battling against the people of the light.”

We went to the Spy Post military base and picked up Major Morris who gave me the cup. He got into the front passenger seat.

“Our lives are at stake Frederick.” said Samantha worriedly. “Here are your D-Day papers. You win this one and you are free for ever.” She said hugging me.

Peter drove the jeep along the motorway to Salisbury Plain. Samantha told me I had no fewer than five hundred highly trained soldiers at my disposal. We would be meeting General Thomson and the troops. Even members of the British Secret Air Service will take part with other cracked troops. Luckily the base above ground was still under our control.

As we drove I felt sick, but it was so urgent we could not stop. Then I went to sleep and rested my head on Samantha's shoulder. I was woken up when the jeep stopped.

"We have arrived." announced Samantha. "Its show time Frederick."

We went into the base and were greeted by General Thomson. He regretted that I was sick, but we had to go to work immediately. He explained to me that I had to lead his troops into battle. We then drove far into the base and the troops came into view. Peter stopped the jeep, and the general commanded the troops with a military briefing.

I listened as the general read the D-Day papers and there was a huge cheer.

"Let them have it boys!" shouted the general, and everybody was ready to make battle against the dreaded Nazi's. "Yours is the hour of Glory!"

Samantha came up to me and gave me a uniform and a beret.

“You qualify to join my ranks any day!” She commanded. “Put it on Private Pucklesquash. I put on the small uniform and it fitted. “How do you feel Frederick?”

“I am ready for D-Day.” I replied and the sergeant saluted me and handed me the cup.

I drank from the cup and looked into the ruby.” Apollyon? Apollyon?” I cried as I shone brilliant white.

“Rely on me Private Pucklesquash.” came Apollyon chuckle. “This is the hour of light when most surely there will be no shadow left in the land.”

The soldiers were amazed and it built up their confidence.

“Trust in your heart Private Pucklesquash.” said the general.

“Private Pucklesquash at your service sir.” I replied saluting.

“Let D-Day commence!” bellowed the general and suddenly dozens of missile silos were opened.

The Nazi's blocked our usual way through the tunnel, but there are many ways to cook an egg. Samantha, Peter, Major Morris, General Thomson, the troops and I descended the ropes. Suddenly there was sporadic gun fire. We got to the bottom. The gunfire intensified and a couple of our men were shot. I drank from the cup and I shone brilliant white. This scared the Nazi's and they began to retreat.

Shots came my direction but could not hit me, whilst Samantha and Peter ducked out of the way and returned fire. Our men were already arresting the Nazi's and leaving the dead. I held my cup high and cried "Apollyon? Apollyon?" and the guns of the Nazi's in the missile chamber jammed. Now we could get access to the city. The general left a couple dozen men to secure our exit as we marched on to the city.

"Come on Private. Left, right, left, right!" said Peter grinning, as I held the cup above my head. I was leading the troops.

We fought from chamber to chamber. Several Nazi's were shot dead. Our fatalities were kept to the minimum. We fought our way out of the missile zone and soon reached the city.

Many Nazi's were shot and we lost more men. However, our troops were highly trained and were a match for the troops of darkness. Peter and Samantha did their best to protect me and every time I cried "Apollyon? Apollyon?" the Nazi's rifles would jam.

A slave girl walked up to me, fumbled around in her rag garment and handed me a worn out book. I looked at the front cover and just made out the words "New Testament".

"You have come at last." She smiled from ear to ear. "You have come!" she said hugging me with delight. "I want to see the sun and green grass!"

The slaves then turned on the guards and began beating them. Our soldiers did not intervene. They had their chance to make peace but they had blown it.

"Well done Frederick!" said Samantha, crying as she hugged me. Even Peter hugged me.

The underground came to a standstill as many wanted to come up to me and thank me and my soldiers.

"Freedom!" I shouted and gazed about and the crowd began to chant "Freedom". Freedom!"

I had tears in my eyes and now it was my job to lead the slaves out of the underground to the base on top. They were at last free. We began to march; the slaves came up and just wanted to touch me. They kept on shaking my hand and giving me bits of food. This was a generous thing to do as they were starved. They trusted in me. I was very emotional as they began telling me about the persecution. They had lost parents, sibling and children. Now they were free. I cried and felt it was a great privilege for me to work for the forces of light.

Suddenly there was a cry and the slaves ran back to their positions. I looked around and saw three men in black cloaks. They stood in a line and unveiled themselves. Each was holding a silver cup with a black stone and on their chest was the number 6. When they stood in a line, it read 666 - The number of the beast of Babylon. They drank from the cups and suddenly out of their mouths wafted smoke. One of them drew a pistol.

“Nobody will help you now son of the light!” said their leader. “You are weaker than us!”

I held my cup to my lips, but they shot it out of my hand and it ended up on the floor with the contents splashed our in front of me.

“Do you wish to join us, Son of God?.” grinned another picking up my cup.

“No never!” I replied.

“We will make you a general!” another replied.

“No never!” I replied.

“We will give you the authority to rule with us, Son of God!”

“No never!” I replied and the army opened fire but none of the bullets struck them.

`Very well.” replied the leader.” Then DIE!”

They opened fire and I was struck all over. I fell to my knees and Samantha screamed. They shot me to pieces and my uniform was covered in blood. I collapsed forward onto the wet surface made by the contents of my cup. Samantha and Peter rushed to me.

“Your troops will be our slaves!” said the leading demon cupbearer and disarmed the general. `The devil looks after his own!” He grinned revealing a black set of teeth.

I felt the wine enter my wound and suddenly I began to shine. I slowly got on my knees to the disbelief of the sons of Satan. The wounds suddenly healed and there wasn’t even a mark on me apart from bullet marks in my clothes. The slaves came closer and starred in astonishment.

“Apollyon! Apollyon! Apollyon!” I bellowed as loud as I could.

The cup flew from the demon cupbearer leader and straight into my hands. I drank from the cup and I glowed more intense than I ever did.

“FREEDOM!” I bellowed.” FREEDOM!”

The slaves seeing this began to chant with me. Suddenly the machines ground to a halt and the light flickered off. Everybody gasped. The emergency lights came on as the computers exploded and caught fire setting off the sprinklers.

The demon cupbearers looked at me in astonishment. There was a loud hissing noise and booming coming from the cup. It was deafening and suddenly parts of the ceiling started caving in. The slaves ran to the exit with everybody else. Just the demon cupbearers, Peter, Samantha, Major Morris and the general stood there. Suddenly fork lightening came out of my cup and electrocuted the three lords of darkness. Then it became so intense that they screamed and collapsed to the floor and disappeared. Just their black cloaks and the three cups were left.

“That’s another three.” said Major Morris picking up the cup.

One Nazi came back and handed me his rifle. “My soldiering days are over!” he spoke. I nodded. “Bravo!” He saluted.

We led the rest of the slaves out of the murky dark dank base to the sunshine above.

“What is that light in the sky?” asked one slave boy.

“That is the sun.” I said biting my lip.

Peter and Samantha drove me back after the General said he’d liked to promote me. I grinned at him. I took my uniform off and became Frederick Pucklesquash again. Now I would be released at last.

Chapter Fifteen

A different branch of the MOD ordered Samantha and Peter to experiment on me. So they would often come and dope me and take me to the local underground listening post on the hills. They even experimented on Apollyon's cup. They experimented on me until I was fifteen. Because of the constant doping I was eventually not able to recognise Sergeant Smith or Peter unless I was doped again, as the drug caused a loss in memory. I was suffering severe amnesia.

I went all through the years of school not knowing that I was drugged by the MOD. I was given plenty of written tests and sent for X-rays at the hands of the MOD. I would basically function normally under the influence of the drug but when they wore off I would not be able to remember a thing unless the drug was injected into the blood stream again. Slowly through the experiments new drugs were designed and I acted as a human guinea pig.

Another reason for the MOD carrying on with drugging me was to design a drug where they could kidnap a foreign spy, drug him, question him without his knowing as no knowledge was retained after the antidote was given. This is how the MOD caught spies and gained highly sensitive information from foreign sources.

I was often sick and missed lot of days off school because the drugs were having an adverse affect on me. I became confused, exhausted, depressed, manic, and hyperactive. Fatigue and tiredness became a problem.

Samantha and Peter thought it would be good for me to have a bit of enjoyable recreation and so they took me to the underground to a nightclub. When we drove back to my home we sat in the back of the jeep chatting. Our meetings became more and more frequent. But this was not to last. Samantha was becoming more distraught and irritated. We desperately wanted a way out but under such circumstances it was impossible. Unless I was given the drug I would not even remember them.

One night we were at an underground base when I passed out. Samantha bellowed for an ambulance. Once it arrived, the paramedics picked me up off the floor and moved me by stretcher into the ambulance. Samantha got in next to me.

"Please God don't let him die!" cried Samantha.

"Just calm down sergeant." was the reply of the paramedic. "He is just exhausted."

"Friedrich, can you hear me?" Peter said putting a hand on my shoulder to reassure me.

If I died there and then, all the police would do is put me on the missing list, like so many others that became comatic due to the drugs that the MOD injected them with.

We soon arrived at the underground hospital and Peter faithfully followed with his jeep. The underground police escorted us. All I could say was "Apollyon, don't let me die!" Over and over again. I was soon given oxygen and Samantha held my hand.

"Come on Friedrich. Don't give up!" whispered Samantha. "I'm not going to give up on you, so don't give up on me." I was given a tranquilliser and after a short while I came around to Samantha's great relief. She was at the end of her nerves and cried bitterly.

"It's all my fault. I will never forgive myself for letting them experiment on you."

However, she was taking orders from her superiors and the experiments were compulsory. She had no say in this.

"You know, from our records he could die if you continue with the experiment. He is going to be psychotic for the rest of his life anyway." said the doctor.

"Oh no! I don't want to know!" replied Samantha. "This is just a complete nightmare."

“Unfortunately that is the legacy of working with the MOD.” said the doctor pausing and rubbing his chin with one hand. “I have seen this happen many times.”

The doctor walked away, leaving Samantha in despair. I was soon discharged. Peter drove us to my home. Samantha worried all the way. I thought she was going to have a nervous breakdown.

“If only they would finish the experiments.” said Samantha.

“My sentiments exactly.” replied Peter sadly. “We did not know the drugs would do this to you son. “

I was more like a son to Samantha and she was like a mother to me. We said our goodbyes, and I felt that Samantha had really become unstable. Over the recent months her mood had changed. She really desired me to be free but her superiors treated me as if I were another statistic. She had been on antidepressants for a couple of months. She became really sad.

I felt sorry for her but I somehow knew we were never going to see each other again. We hugged for the last time. I asked Peter to look after her, but all he could do was shake my hand and give me a watery smile. When I walked away I somehow already felt that we were walking away from each other forever. It was the saddest day of my life.

Chapter Sixteen

One morning I was on my way to school, which was about a mile and a half walk to the bus stop from our bungalow. As I was walking down the country lanes under the big oaks and the conker trees that were dripping from the rain, I stepped into a puddle by accident. I bent down to tie up my boot when a military truck pulled up. Men jumped out and injected me with serum and helped me up onto the back of the truck. They closed the back but there was a light and I could see Peter's distraught face.

"I am very sorry Friedrich." he said in a sad voice and handed me a letter as the truck pulled off and made its way to the local army base. The letter was addressed to me. I felt sick and anxious. It read: -

Dear Friedrich,

I can no longer live with the idea that we experimented with you and made you so ill. I am consumed by guilt. I have had a nervous breakdown. How Could I have done all this to somebody so innocent? I am in the lap of the Gods. Perhaps Apollyon will have mercy on my soul.

Please forgive me for doing this, but I can no longer live and be happy while you have to suffer so horrendously. I am leaving a lot of people behind, but I can't help it. I have felt suicidal for weeks. There is no way out.

Please forgive me.

Yours

Samantha

I cried as I read the letter. Through eyes streaming with tears I turned to Peter.

"Is she dead?" I asked.

"I am afraid so." replied Peter sadly, and lit up a cigarette. "I am ever so sorry. She meant a lot to both of us."

I cried and felt shocked. It was frightening to lose a close friend. I just imagine her not being there for me any more. I tasted the salt from my tears in my mouth. I put my head in my hands and howled. It was just so sad. Why the hell did she have to go through with it? I started going through the "If only's" and I just muttered to myself. I was devastated.

I was driven to the lab on the underground and I was injected with a newly developed drug. The drug, in time, would help me to remember all the other times I had been drugged and it would become part of my conscious mind. I was then released and that was the last time I went into the underground. Peter hoped that one day I would sue the MOD. Peter tearfully said goodbye to me, gave me an antidote and I forgot everything.

It was not until I was nineteen, four years later, that I remembered Samantha. Everything started coming back to me but nobody believed me. I became more and more depressed and confused. I felt tormented by the injustice but absolutely nobody would believe me. I hated the MOD for what they did to Sergeant Smith. She desperately needed psychotherapy. I realised I could not live this way with such troubling thoughts. I took my penknife and went out in the middle of a farm field on top of the hill and sat down. I began a silent prayer.

"No young man this is not the way of a hero." came a gentle, voice as a hand grabbed my hand in which I held the knife.

I stared up from my sitting position and I saw a person I thought I would never see again.

"Hello... so it is true after all...Hello Apollyon." I said with tears in my eyes and then I Looked behind me and saw the carriage.

"I have a friend to see you."

"I'm glad to see you. I am fed up with life."

“Perhaps I can cheer you up.” replied Apollyon with a chuckle. “Have a look in my carriage.”

I got up off the ground and accompanied Apollyon to the carriage. He opened the carriage door and within sat a female angel beaming at me. I saw her soft feathers and that familiar expression of affection on her face. I stared in utter amazement. I slowly got up in the carriage.

“But . . ., but . . ., well . . . , what the . . . ? “ I was speechless and dumb struck as I saw the angel with that familiar twinkle in her dark brown eyes. “ SAMANTHA! It’s you!”

“Hello Friedrich.” she said and we threw ourselves in each other’s arms. “Oh Friedrich I’ve missed you.”

“Samantha, you’re alive!”

We hugged as Apollyon threw back his head and laughed. The heavens opened and a wonderful sound came from an orchestra of angels. I was the Messiah that had freed the slaves and caused the end of the cold war, which in time will be realised.

I was so happy to see Samantha again. The angels applauded, and Samantha and I stayed in each other’s arms and cried for joy.

From now on Samantha was to become my guardian angel. Never again do I have to feel lonely. Sometimes, I can feel her touch, her soft warm wings around me and I can hear her gentle voice in my ear. Wherever I went, wherever I stayed, whenever I was alone she would be there comforting me with her presence and whispering softly in my ear.

Chapter Seventeen

Dr. Bolger had patiently listened to me all this time. I felt that perhaps sometimes she was amused but on other occasions she was quite amazed at my bizarre thoughts. One minute I felt elated and the next I felt depressed. I always wanted to write a book on my bizarre thoughts.

"Do you believe in all what you told me Friedrich?" she asked.

"It's gospel true." I replied.

"Can you still hear Samantha's voice?"

"Yes I can."

"When do you hear them?"

"When I am depressed and my thoughts rush around and my mind is hyperactive."

"What does she say?"

"She gives me a lot of comforting messages and then I feel warm. Sometimes I imagine I am on the underground with her and we are driving in the jeep."

"Well Friedrich, you are quite sick. You believe that your fantasies are a reality. You have a psychosis and the voice you hear is a hallucination."

"The doctor on the underground said that I was psychotic." I replied.

"We are going to take some samples from you. Will you give us your written permission to treat you by signing a form?"

"If it means I don't have to suffer so much."

"Have you taken any drugs recently?"

"The only drugs I take are coffee and nicotine." I replied in a half joking sort of way. "Do you think I am a messiah who freed the slaves?"

"You don't smoke cannabis or take drugs like LSD or amphetamines?" she asked ignoring my question.

"I don't take any drugs apart from coffee, cider and nicotine."

I paused for a while as my head was buzzing with ideas. My mind was so hyperactive that I could hardly sleep.

"What does your doctor say about your illness?"

"He says I have got hypomania." I replied pausing. "Are you sure I'm ill and not a chosen one?

“You have a very active mind and a fertile imagination. It does seem to me that you are suffering from schizophrenia.”

“Schizophrenia?” I asked horrified. “Is it curable?”

“Something can be done about it. We may put you on an injection later but until then refrain from taking any medication. We don’t want you to leave the hospital for a home visit for two weeks. Then you can have weekend leave.”

That finished my appointment with Dr. Bolger. After a few more interviews I was given a diagnosis of schizophrenia by the medical team. So at long last I was given the proper treatment. I stayed in hospital for six weeks and then they discharged me. I had had a schizophrenic breakdown and it would take a couple of years to recover from some of the symptoms but the worst of the hallucinations abated within days.

My mind slowed down and for a change I could sleep again. The bizarre fantasies abated but not totally until a few years after. But I was capable of living with my family again.

After six weeks I was released and my mind felt more normal again.

I used to sleep a lot as the tranquillizers made me drowsy. They often caused me to drift off.

I woke up one day and went down stairs for a coffee. The doorbell rang. I went to the front door and opened it.

“Hello, I just wondered if you would like your milk delivered?” said a familiar man with flame red hair, pop eyes and a scar across his face.

His smile made him look friendlier; or at least less frightening.

“Rather you do these early mornings than me.” I replied chuckling.

“I’m used to it.” he replied smiling.” I had many early mornings in the army.”

“Where were you stationed?” I asked awkwardly.

“In Detmold, Germany.” he replied.

I slammed the door shut and rushed into the kitchen.

“What’s a matter dear?” asked my mother grinning.

“I’m hallucinating!” I replied grabbing my pills and a cup of water.

“You met Alf the milkman did you?” she asked.

`Yes." I replied. "The man with the scar and pop eyes."

`Don't worry, he is very friendly." she smiled and chuckled and walked out.

THE END

www.ingramcontent.com/pod-product-compliance
Lightning Source LLC
LaVergne TN
LVHW090953080826
845145LV00003B/996

* 9 7 8 1 8 4 7 4 7 1 1 2 3 *